ECZEMA DECODED

ECZEMA
decoded

How to Rescue
Yourself and Your Children
from Atopic Dermatitis

CAROLYN AKINYEMI

Copyright 2021 Carolyn Akinyemi

Typesetting and cover design:
Joanna & Grzegorz Japoł - LUNA Design Studio

ISBN: 978-1-9996996-3-5

The author of this book does not dispense any medical advice or prescribe the use of any medications or forms of treatment for Eczema. The intention of the author is merely to offer information to help you in your own quest for healing and for you to share with your medical practitioner as you work with them under their guidance. Should you choose to action the information in this book without seeking medical guidance, the author accepts no responsibility for your actions.

This book is dedicated to Esther, Rebecca, Hannah and Isaiah, my beloved children who were caught in the eczema spider web for so many years. You endured not just the pain and suffering of eczema (even though that is no small thing) but also the atopic march and my persistent experimentations of many different solutions and remedies as I refused to accept defeat, always believing there had to be more to this than I was being told. I love you all immensely. This is as much your story as mine, as we have fought this eczema battle together.

I also want to thank Ayoola for your support while I focused my energies on writing this book. I am very grateful for your encouragement throughout this project.

And finally, I want to include all the warriors who have stoically endured the torment of eczema and to your loved ones who are desperately seeking to discover the best ways to help you! You were my inspiration to write down and publish everything I had learned. **I understand what you are going though, and I care. I feel your frustration. I've lived the struggle. You are not alone. There is hope! This book is for you.**

Contents

SECTION 1:

Caught In The Spider Web

Introduction

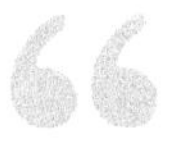 *Any fool can make something complicated. It takes a genius to make it simple".*

Woody Guthrie

The dictionary definition of the word '*decoded*' means to convert into intelligible language, to analyze and interpret a communication, or to convert something into a different or usable form.

Whilst I am not near genius in my abilities, it IS my intention to decode the complicated maze of eczema healing and present it in a way that is both simple to understand and easy to action. To achieve this, I have endeavoured to convert scientific research papers on the treatment of eczema into lay terms for the understanding of those who do not possess a medical degree but require the information contained within them. I hope I have successfully achieved this to help the millions of you who are continually frustrated by the lack of real explanation as to why you have eczema and how you can find healing. I pray that you, the reader, find your answers in these pages. If this is the case, please help others by leaving a positive review on Amazon; this will help the book to be more prominently listed in search results and help others to find it.

You can also subscribe to my channel and view my videos at

The Eczema Channel - YouTube

1

The Billion Dollar Question

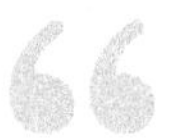 *Would it make good business sense to manufacture a product that actually cures eczema?"*

That was the ominous question that gatecrashed my mind unexpectedly, and at that moment, with a small mountain of emollient cream in my hand, I froze. I was about to compliantly slather my baby girl with the prescribed treatment for her eczema; however, suddenly, I was unable to do it. I felt sick. Would somebody really want to profit from my baby's suffering?

I was unaware of it at the time, but that one little question had just hugely impacted my life, like a meteor knocking a cosmic body off its trajectory! The haunting implications of that suggestion increased exponentially when I had three more children in close succession, with every one of them developing eczema. Parenting children is an immensely challenging role, even under normal circumstances. However, when you add in eczema, wet wraps, emollient creaming multiple times a day, applying topical steroids, trying desperately to find ways to relieve that tormenting itching and consequent scratching, and then negotiating the subsequent allergies that manifest as part of the atopic march, it quickly becomes an all-consuming full-time job. Now multiply that by four, and you will have a glimpse at my early motherhood experience. By that point, I was reading every ingredient in the pharmaceutical treatments and google searching to determine exactly what they were and how they worked. Ultimately, that seemingly innocuous question sparked the beginning of years of research into the mechanisms of eczema and discoveries that would never have been made without that prompt. Thus, let us think about that question for a moment.

From a business model point of view, a company that produces a cure for a disease will reap immediate profits. Their cure will become widely known as healed patients shout from the rooftops about the wonders of this treatment. But what are the long-term results for the company? Well, as a consequence, they will subsequently lose all of their customers in that niche. In fact, as people are healed, their client base will decline until they no longer have a viable market. Furthermore, once patients are cured, they no longer need the products purported to treat the disease. As corrupt as it sounds, there is simply no financial benefit to the company in healing you or your children entirely of any chronic illness, not just eczema. It would be much more viable to manufacture products that can temporarily alleviate symptoms but which…well, maybe…contain ingredients that help to perpetuate the problem, resulting in customers that stay dependent on those products for the rest of their lives. Look at this sentence I am quoting from the website of a medical institution: "Because these (talking about eczema and psoriasis) are chronic inflammatory skin conditions, these clients can be a valuable business opportunity, with an increased likelihood of return bookings." My heart was grieved when I read this. To see organizations viewing eczema patients (like you and your children) as great business opportunities or cash cows to be utilized for financial gain really upsets me. These are real people with real pain who need real help!

This whole theory could be over suspicion on my part. Some may say I have read too many conspiracy theory novels in the past, or my protective motherly instinct had run off track somewhere and was now jumping over hurdles that were not in my lane. Either way, I determined I would not just nod my head, acquiesce and let my babies get caught in anyone's gravy train without first researching for myself. So that was how my Eczemalogy™ Map began.

Anyone impacted by eczema, either themselves or who has watched loved ones suffer, knows that it is a heart-breaking condition. There is not only that constant tormenting itch that defies all attempts to block it but also the cosmetic appearance of the eczema rash, which too often causes embarrassment and rejection in public. "It is not contagious. It's eczema," you say as a mother pulls her young child away from yours. "No, you cannot catch it from being close to my child," you reassure another, and your heart breaks each time your child is looked at warily as if they were a leper who had escaped quarantine.

It affects me deeply when I see children and babies covered in eczema. They live with a far higher stress level than they ought to due to the constant physical symptoms, yet they cannot express their feelings. This can cause feelings of injustice to develop as they wonder why they are tormented by endless itching and prickling when other children play happily, unaffected, and perfectly comfortable in their skin. For adults and children alike, the pain and discomfort resulting from eczema lesions can seriously affect the ability to sleep and focus on daily tasks, whether at work, school, or play. This is without mentioning the frustration and feelings of hopelessness and despair when eczema flares up repeatedly for no known reason, despite everything you try. Your mind is bombarded with questions. Why did my child get this? Did I do anything wrong? Is it hereditary? Is there anything I can use to improve it? Can I stop it from spreading? How do I stop that constant itching and prickling? Will anything help me get a better night's sleep? Why does it seem to improve and then flare up again? What are the side effects of the treatment options? How can I focus better on work or school? When will I get healed from this? Will I EVER get healed? Who can I turn to for real answers?

In 'Eczema Decoded', I aim to answer all the above questions and more. To pre-empt your question, "Who am I and what qualifies me to teach people about eczema?" I will answer honestly; I am not a doctor, nor do I have any medical degrees. However, I have researched eczema extensively for over 10 years, studying peer-reviewed scientific papers in various academic fields and desperately searching for answers to help my four children break free from eczema. I used to believe that no one would listen to me due to my lack of formal medical training. Still, I now realize that this has helped me discover the extensive information that benefitted my mission. Not having one line of discipline in my studies means I have not been blinkered in my research, which I may have been had I been enrolled in a university course that focused on just one discipline or field of study. In addition, I have not been trained in the doctrine of Big Pharma. Your medical professional will tell you that eczema is incurable because that is what they have been taught in their pharma-sponsored medical training. They are taught that eczema is for life and to prescribe treatments to manage the symptoms, often at the risk of developing undesirable side effects. They can only teach what they know from their training. In contrast, I have gained deep knowledge through broad-reaching, independent research, and personal experience helping my family and others.

One of my mantras is, "Desperate mums do amazing things!" I was a desperate mum; from the moment my first child developed eczema at only eight weeks old, something in me refused to accept that this was just the result of an inherited weakness or, as we were told, "Oh, you have an atopic family." I did not know what to do about my daughter's condition and trusted that our family doctors would have the expertise and knowledge to teach us how to heal her. However, I soon realized that the standard protocol that eczema patients are told to follow is not a path to healing but rather one of symptom management. If your life has been impacted by eczema, I know you will be thinking, as I did, there must be a better way than this. Well, I am happy to tell you that there is. I will not give you soundbites or contradictory surface-level opinions from search engines. Instead, I will share with you real, evidenced, peer-reviewed, actionable protocols I have gathered from international research documents. I used it to heal my own four children (and myself after I developed eczema on my hands, aged in my forties). It works; therefore, figuratively speaking, take my hand and let me walk you on a guided tour through this maze called eczema.

When I teach people in person, or as happens more often now, on Zoom, I treat eczema like an onion, peeling back various layers one at a time. I do this for two reasons; firstly, to bring suggestions for external relief as quickly as possible, and secondly, because the roots are easier to understand when they are exposed one by one. By teaching this way, I help people understand what is happening inside their bodies, which empowers them to take corrective action both now and in the future. If they ever 'fall off the wagon,' so to speak, they will have the tools to get back on it again. In my opinion, that is a much better solution than making people dependent, telling them things to try but no reasons why, and having them return for more medication or products time and time again.

I will follow the same pattern in this book, peeling back the layers one at a time and showing the 'why' and the 'what' to empower you to understand the workings of eczema inside your body and to take action to correct it. Desmond Tutu once said: "How do you eat an elephant? One bite at a time!" The saying makes a good point; you can accomplish seemingly insurmountable tasks if they are tackled in smaller pieces. Similarly, if you ask me, "How do you escape chronic eczema?" My answer would be "By dealing with one layer at a time."

Now, before we start peeling your onion, we first need to expose the biggest myth there is regarding eczema. Are you ready for this?

2

Busting The Biggest Myth

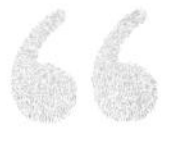

*The reason why you have been told there is no cure
for eczema is because eczema is NOT
what is wrong with you!"*

When you initially received the diagnosis of eczema, if you were like me, you simultaneously felt both horror that your baby (or you) had what is believed to be an incurable disease, and relief that your doctor has identified what is wrong and how to manage it. Then, you embark enthusiastically on the protocol of treatments I spoke about in the previous chapter. Your mission is to break free from this horrid condition; however, it then begins to dawn on you that you are walking on a road of frustration, constantly battling re-occurring flare-ups, and you cannot fathom why it keeps coming back and is indeed relentlessly spreading.

I am going to burst the bubble and expose what I believe is the biggest myth about eczema out there. The myth is that there is a disease called eczema. Yes, you read that correctly. The biggest myth that has people going around in circles looking for a non-existent cure is that there is even a disease called eczema at all. Some may think I am crazy for saying this, but please hear me out. The reason why you have been told there is no cure for eczema is because eczema is NOT what is wrong with you. Eczema is not a disease; it is merely the label that best describes your set of symptoms. Even the definition of eczema in the Medical Dictionary confirms this. I quote:

"Eczema: *any superficial inflammatory process involving primarily the epidermis,* marked early by redness, itching, minute papules and vesicles, weeping, oozing, and crusting, and later by scaling, lichenification, and often pigmentation." (Italics added for emphasis)

Do you notice that a diagnosis of eczema is given to any superficial inflammatory process involving the upper skin layer (epidermis), so long as it manifests the type of symptoms listed? Thus, being told that you have eczema just means your symptoms have been given a label; however, it does not mean that anyone has investigated what has actually gone wrong inside you to cause these symptoms or subsequently diagnosed what is really wrong with you and how to put it right.

Let me repeat my statement even more loudly. Excuse me for shouting, but it is vital for you to grasp this. "ECZEMA IS NOT WHAT IS WRONG WITH YOU. IT IS JUST THE LABEL THAT BEST DESCRIBES YOUR SET OF SYMPTOMS." So far, no one has told you what is wrong with you. Let me explain further.

Humans tend to categorize things into boxes to determine where everything fits in life and where we fit in comparison. It makes us feel secure and makes life easier to negotiate and manage. For example, we talk about home life, work life, and social life, and we break the week into workdays and weekends. A good example is the way we label colours into categories, including blue shades, red shades, and so on, whereas colour is instead a continual spectrum; it does not occur in the simple categories or boxes we give to it. We do this because it makes it easier for us to talk about them and work with them. Furthermore, we compartmentalize society by demographics and geographical areas by boroughs, cities, towns, and wards, whereas in reality, urban neighbourhoods flow into each other without any physical barriers to show where the boundary lines lie. Other examples are science, which is divided into different 'ologies,' and food, which is divided into carbohydrates, proteins, fats, and macro and micronutrients. However, food items are not a source of just one sole nutrient but instead a blend of many varied composites in the nutritional spectrum. For example, we tend to view meat as protein, but it also contains fat, which can be a great energy source, along with iron and vitamin B12. Nuts are considered a high source of fat, but they also contain proteins and carbohydrates, along with magnesium and other nutrients.

We chronicle events by time periods, and even the books we read are divided by chapter and paragraph. Why do we do this? Compartmentalizing everything enables our brains to sort life into manageable, organized chunks, whether it is social, business, employment, education, or health. It also allows us to 'grade' ourselves against others and see where we 'fit' in the grand scheme of things. For example, are we upper, middle, or working class? Are we educated to High School, College, or Degree level? How do we compare to our family members or our neighbours?

The medical model we currently adhere to also functions by using this categorization model, and as such, we have divided medicine into specialities. We have cardiology, endocrinology, dermatology, orthopaedics, psychiatry, and gastroenterology, to name only a few. The downside of this approach is that the medical profession has divided the body into sections or systems. Consequently, it has proceeded to treat the body as if a disease is somehow limited to being in only that area or system. Conditions are then 'identified' by applying a label, sort of like an umbrella term, under which a group of common symptoms are listed. By determining which umbrella a patient can be categorized under, a medical professional can then prescribe the drugs to treat (which really could be more accurately called 'mask' or 'manage') the symptoms that are associated with that label. That is the process of diagnosis that we use today. However, let me ask you a couple of questions. Has anyone explicitly identified what is wrong with you? Has anyone told you what made those symptoms manifest in the first place? How about pinpointing the root cause of the problem? No, I suspect not. Only the symptom label you fit under has likely been identified so that you can be prescribed the appropriate drugs or pharmaceutical interventions to manage those symptoms. In the case of eczema, it is a label that covers symptoms such as dry, itchy skin, patches of inflammation, rough, leathery, or scaly areas of skin, small blisters that can be filled with fluid, and areas of oozing and crusting.

This is why you are told there is no cure for eczema; eczema is not the diagnosis of what has gone wrong inside your body. It is only the disease label that you have been placed under. Hence why, you have not been healed. You cannot be cured of a label. This is the same for any chronic medical condition. The current medical model is not a system of healing or health care. It is instead a system of symptom management. Medics are taught to identify symptoms and prescribe pharmaceutical 'remedies' to manage those symptoms. However, no one can be healed from a label because a label is not a disease. To be healed, you must first determine what is wrong with you, which involves finding the root cause of your symptoms.

Disease in our bodies is rather like disease in a tree. If you had a lovely fruit tree that suddenly began to bear abnormal-looking fruit, you may initially pull off those few fruits, throw them away, and hope the new ones grow back better. However, if the tree continues to produce unhealthy fruit and the problem worsens, you will have a choice. You could persist in doing the same things you have already done and continue reaping the same futile results, or you can look beyond the fruit and investigate what might be wrong with the tree itself. There could be a fungal or parasite infection, a problem with the soil or climate, or even an undiscovered issue with roots.

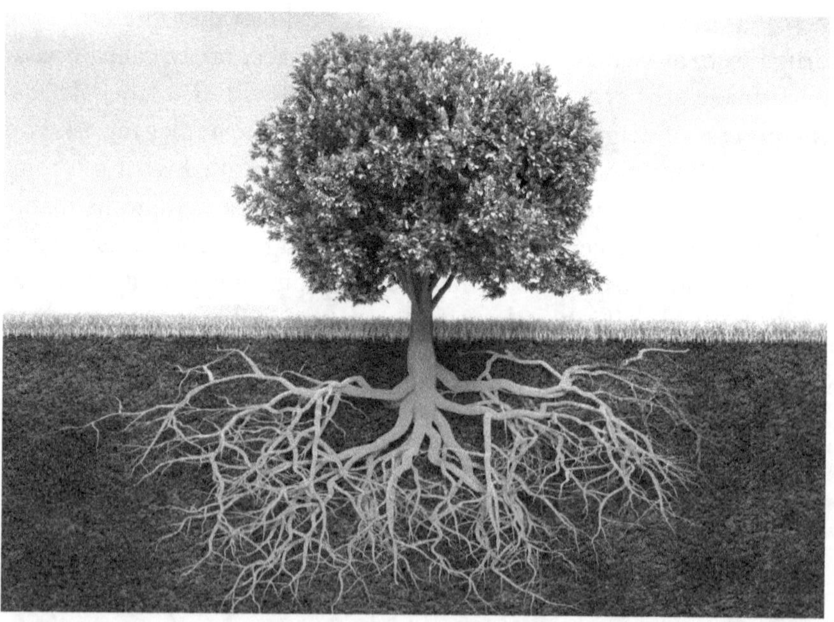

The tree in the picture above reminds me very much of eczema. Although the disease symptoms may be seen on the surface, the root of the problem lies way below ground level and often become entangled with other issues that require some detective work to unravel.

With that premise in mind, we must change how we view two things to determine the root causes of eczema. Firstly, ourselves, and secondly, whose responsibility it is for our healing and well-being.

Our body is not a collection of individual systems that just happen to co-exist inside us. It is one intertwined unit, functioning as a whole system. Remember, every part of our body grew from the same fertilized egg, which continued to divide, multiply, and adapt until it created all the complexities of our human form, neatly wrapped within our envelope of skin. In fact, because the skin is part of this fantastic interdependent unit, it can manifest as a reflection of what is going on inside our body. It does not cooperate with the independent 'dermatology category designated by the medical profession. It is one part of an intricately designed, interdependent unit, just like the tree above. Thus, if the skin is not functioning optimally, an internal issue most likely needs to be addressed. This is what your body is calling your attention to.

When your baby feels discomfort, pain, fear, or is unwell, its main course of action to get your attention is to fuss and cry to let you know something is amiss. As a devoted parent, you will attend to your child's cries, and often by process of elimination (especially in the early days), you will try to identify the problem. You do not expect your baby to eloquently tell you precisely what the issue is; it does not have the ability to do so and consequently uses the only means it has at its disposal – crying. Your body is very much like your baby because it uses the means at its disposal to tell you something is amiss. That means is often disease, which functional and integrative type doctors will tell you is really dis-ease, meaning the body is not at ease. Therefore, when that happens, we have to investigate, with the same attentiveness and care that we give to our children when they cry, what is causing the issue. Just as you should not gag a crying baby, you should also not try to gag your body with pharmaceutical band-aids when it is crying for help. Dis-ease should not be suppressed but addressed. If you do not help it, your body will invariably start to cry even louder in the form of more symptoms, leading to more labels and pharmaceutical medications with more side effects. It is a downward spiralling helter-skelter ride; however, rather than being a fun fairground ride, it is a black hole that can take us far from health and wellness.

This leads me to the second change in point of view: whose responsibility is it to look after your health and well-being? Who should be responsible for finding out what exactly is wrong with you? Is it the National Health Service? Your medical insurance company? Your government? If you believe this to be so, I apologize for sounding harsh, but you need to stop expecting other people to spoon-feed you. It is time for you to start taking responsibility for your life, your health, and the decisions that have led you here. Disease does not just happen. There is always at least one reason. You must discover these reasons, whether it is your diet, poor stress management, exposure to toxins, or any other number of issues, and then start to put it right. I once heard someone say that Big Pharma has about as much interest in you achieving optimal health as arms (weapons) manufacturing companies have in world peace. If you get healed, they lose money. It is that simple. Hippocrates, widely considered the father of medicine, said, "Before you heal anyone, ask him if he is ready to give up the things that made him sick." You need to ask yourself this question. There may be things in your environment, foods you love, and habits you have become accustomed to that are contributing to your disease. Are you ready to give them up if we identify them as making you sick? The answer is not an obvious one. Believe it or not, some people would rather not make those uncomfortable decisions and would prefer to stay chronically ill. Therefore, let us get clear on this issue before we go any further. No one else is responsible for your health and wellness apart from YOU. Are YOU ready to give up the things that are making you sick? Yes, I understand we are not always responsible for what happens to us in life, what toxins we have been exposed to, what mistakes others have made, and so on. However, it IS our responsibility to choose how we respond to those circumstances.

Once I realized this, my 'mamma lion' instinct kicked in, and I started to fight. I set a goal to identify the root cause of my children's eczema and find safe symptomatic relief along the way to alleviate their torment as best as possible. I stopped relying on others to do it for me. Having helped my family, I began to help others find the root cause of their symptoms. This book is the same material I teach 1:1 clients or course students, but without the live interaction and questions and answers. (If you would like to find out more about working with me on a personal level, reach out to me on LinkedIn or email me directly: Carolyn@EczemaAcademy.com)

Going back to your eczema situation, would you prefer an accurate diagnosis that identifies the core problem and provides a protocol for addressing the root causes or to stay on the current system of symptom management you are using? Since you are still reading this book, I am assuming that you have decided to take the former rather than the latter option, as you have realized that the path you have been following so far is not getting you where you want to go. Well done. Accepting responsibility for your health is the first hurdle on the track to healing.

The information in this book is not my opinion, nor is it hearsay. It is backed by science. I have spent years researching peer-reviewed science papers and working through online degree modules from various universities in various disciplines in my quest for answers. However, I will confess that I have not found a simple cause and cure that will enable you to see an instant healing trick. If you are looking for a magic wand that will instantly heal eczema, I am sorry to disappoint you; a one-size-fits-all solution simply does not exist. Eczema has taken many years, even generations, to start manifesting, and it will become even more rampant if we continue doing the things that have caused it to develop. I have discovered a tangled web of changes in the body that need to be systematically and individually addressed and untangled. The symptoms labelled as eczema come from a multiple-legged causal creature resembling a giant spider. Its eight legs weave strands of a web that feed into the other legs, perpetuating the condition and making it incredibly challenging to escape without guidance. Eczema can start with one primary cause; however, it quickly becomes a mass of tangled secondary causes, with interconnecting webs that make it difficult to discern where the problem began. Not everyone has the same primary cause, which is why the internet is awash with articles that only work for some. As eczema becomes a chronic condition over time, it creates a cascade of adaptations in the body that help keep the loops immortalized. From personal experience, I know that living with chronic eczema, whether as a patient or the primary caregiver, feels like living with a constant barrage of disappointment; an endless cycle of hope in the latest ideas, and letdowns when they do not work for you, along with the depressive weight of feeling that it is all futile when eczema flares up again and again despite everything you try.

I want to make it clear that although healing eczema is challenging, it is not impossible. Through my research, I identified those eight legs of the eczema spider and mapped the web of what is feeding into what. Armed with that knowledge and my huge Eczemology™ Map, which is placed on the wall in my home, I could disable the legs from feeding into each other and prevent them from eternalizing eczema. This is what I am going to share with you. Once you start to address the primary and secondary root causes of eczema, you can prevent the legs from creating those web strands that perpetuate the disease state and instead begin to heal from within. It is not an instantaneous fix, but once you identify where to start, you can begin to see results surprisingly quickly. Does it take effort on your part? Yes, you have work to do implementing change in your life, but if you have battled with eczema for any length of time, 6-8 weeks will not seem oppressive when you see the improvements week by week. This is not a quick-fix solution. It is a life-changing experience. Some people have experienced clear skin in as little as 28 days, whereas others have taken many months. The truth is the faster you can activate the information in this book, the quicker you can see results. On the bright side, as the spider legs interact with each other a lot, you will find as you progress through this course, tackling each module consequently, you have already actioned a lot of the protocols on previous modules to disable the legs in later modules. Hence, the course has a cumulative effect; the results become exponentially bigger as you implement the action points.

Thus, to find a cure, we must look beyond the symptoms (the diseased fruit on the tree) and delve into what is happening inside (at the roots and in the soil). Below is a simplified visual representation of the eczema spider web with you (or your loved one) trapped in the middle. I am going to teach you, through the rest of this book, about each of these spider legs, how they interact to perpetuate eczema, and how you can disable them naturally.

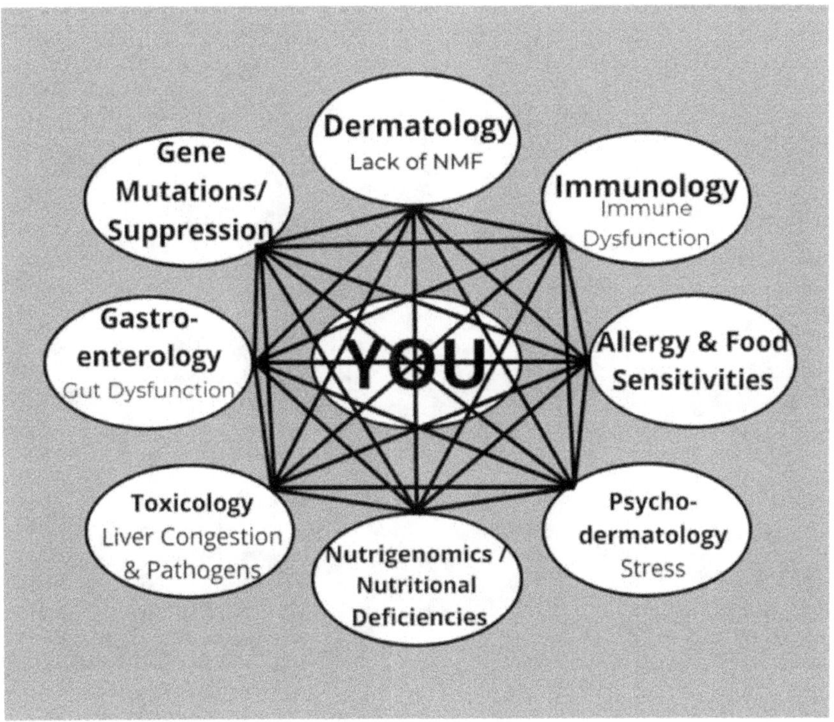

So, are you ready to start your road to recovery? I cannot walk your road for you, but I can be your guide as someone who has travelled this route with all my children and other clients. I cannot force you to action anything I suggest, but in this book, I will teach you how to identify and disable the legs in your own eczema Spider. Before we delve any further though, now that we have established that eczema is a label and not a diagnosis, let me share with you why GETTING OUT from under that eczema umbrella is more urgent than you currently realize.

3

Burdens Beyond the Boundaries

I can still remember the feelings of disbelief, confusion, and exhaustion all landing on me at the same time. I had arrived at the hospital around 10 pm that evening believing I just needed to request some antibiotics for my 7-year-old daughter, who appeared to have a chest infection. Instead, five hours later, at 3 am the next morning, I had a consultant standing before me, telling me she might not even make it.

Around three weeks before this, my daughter contracted a chest infection and was prescribed a short course of antibiotics. She seemed to recover; however, that Sunday, she developed laboured breathing while we were at church and started to develop a fever. My motherly instinct told me that the previous infection had not been cleared and was now attempting to make a come-back. Unfortunately, our doctor's surgery was closed because it was a holiday weekend. Thus, I opted to take her to the Urgent Care Centre at our local hospital, believing I could secure an antibiotic prescription and be on my way.

On arrival, we were seen by the triage nurse, who promptly informed me that my daughter was far too sick to be at Urgent Care because her oxygen levels were too low. She asserted that I should immediately take her to the Pediatric Emergency Department. It was only a short walk along the corridor, but my daughter was quite weak, so I had to carry her. The medics who assessed her decided that as she had both eczema and allergies, she had now developed asthma and was having an Asthma attack. My assurances that she did not suffer from asthma fell on deaf ears, and she was promptly given ten puffs of salbutamol inhaler. Her breathing quickly became easier, to which the nurse declared, "See, I was right. It IS asthma."

I felt confused. This diagnosis did not sit right in my spirit, but the inhaler had worked. Maybe I was wrong.

Less than 20 minutes later, my daughter was struggling to breathe again.

"That is strange", the nurse mused. "It should last longer than 20 minutes." She gave my daughter another ten puffs of salbutamol, which, once again, barely lasted 20 minutes. Her oxygen levels kept falling. I repeatedly asked for a chest X-ray to test for an infection. Finally, after a third dose of ten salbutamol puffs (equating to 30 puffs in just over one hour), she was sent for a chest X-ray, which a doctor examined and declared was clear. My daughter's oxygen levels began dropping again.

"The salbutamol is no longer working. We will have to move to nebulizers," a doctor stated with a concerned look. By now, my daughter was so full of salbutamol that she was shaking terribly, and her heart was racing like a Formula One car. Nebulizers also administer salbutamol through a face mask as a vapour so they are absorbed more effectively. I was torn inside, feeling powerless. I wanted to stop them from giving her even more salbutamol, especially as it did not seem to be working, but I did not understand what was happening or what was wrong with her, and I was scared. These were the qualified medics. Surely, they should know better than me, right?

"Are you sure there are no other options?" I asked anxiously, "Look, she is already shaking so much." I hovered protectively over my daughter, lying weakly on the trolley. The nurse assured me it was just the salbutamol effects and that it would wear off as it came out of her system. She ushered me to the side as she strapped the nebulizer mask around her head. How I hated seeing my little girl like this.

The nebulizers did not work either. With her oxygen levels falling lower, I was told she would be admitted to the hospital and put on intravenous salbutamol. Seeing my daughter in that condition broke my heart, and I felt like I was being railroaded into treatments without understanding why or the side effects. I felt like a failure for not being able to help her or protect her. My gut instinct still told me that this was a chest infection and not an asthma attack, but her oxygen levels were still falling, and her condition was becoming an emergency. I felt that I had to submit to the knowledge of the professionals. They were medically qualified, after all, whereas I was not. Her little face screwed up in pain as the cannula was pushed into the back of her hand for the intravenous tap. She was not even strong enough to fight and gave just a small, pitiful cry.

When we arrived at the ward, she was transferred into the bed, and the nurse placed an oxygen mask over her mouth and nose to help increase her oxygen levels. Worryingly, the intravenous salbutamol sent her heart rate through the roof. Consequently, she was also administered intravenous potassium to replace what the salbutamol was depleting from her system. She was also given intravenous magnesium sulphate solution to relax the muscles in her chest, which led to her vomiting repeatedly as a side effect. The doctors then decided that she needed anti-sickness drugs too because she could not effectively stay on her oxygen mask while continually vomiting.

So, there we were, five hours after we arrived, me exhausted and fraught with anxiety, and my small daughter lying in the hospital bed, with intravenous tubes on both sides, oxygen mask strapped around her head, the heart monitor beeping rapidly to the rhythm of her galloping heart, and the oxygen monitor alarm going off every time she moved and caused her oxygen supply mask to slip.

That was when the consultant arrived and spoke those shocking words, "We do not know which way this is going to go." I had arrived a short time earlier thinking I was coming in for some antibiotics for a chest infection, and now I was being told my daughter might not even make it through the night. She was only seven years old. It goes without saying I did not want to lose her. I called my husband, and he started calling round to mobilise prayer support for our daughter. Shortly after, a nurse came and gave her an injection, and after a while, she began to stabilize.

Towards the end of the night shift, a registrar came by to check on my daughter. He said he had been thinking of her all night and that it did not sit with him that this was the big one, the huge asthma attack that every parent of an asthmatic child dreads. He told me they already know the asthma patients who are at risk of this as they are admitted with many more minor asthmatic episodes long before they have a major event. Then he repeated what I already knew: my daughter had never been to the hospital before with any form of asthma and did not use inhalers at home. The registrar did not offer an alternative explanation but just said he was troubled by it and thought something else was happening. He also told me he found it interesting that she only started to stabilize after she was given hydrocortisone, an anti-inflammatory. I was not even aware that she had been given these steroids, so that was news to me. I assumed it was the injection the nurse had given her.

A few hours later, the primary consultant arrived and started to talk to me about how this was the 'Big One'. It felt like a rehearsed speech he had delivered to many other parents before. However, I interrupted him and said, "Hold on, your registrar was in here just this morning, and he said this…." I proceeded to tell him everything that the register had voiced to me about his concerns. The consultant listened and looked thoughtful for a moment. Then he addressed the original team of doctors and nurses who had attended to my daughter on her arrival in the Emergency Department. They were standing just inside the doorway of the room.

"Did any of you do a chest X-ray?" he asked.

"Yes, we did. It was clear," one of them replied.

The room went silent for a moment. Then the consultant declared, "I want to see it myself." He turned to me and said he would return after he had a chance to review her notes and X-ray.

Later in the day, he returned alone and informed me he had checked the X-ray, and it showed clear indication of a chest infection and a partially collapsed lung! My daughter had been pumped full of unnecessary salbutamol and magnesium sulphate, which required even more drugs to manage the noxious side effects. Yet, all she had needed were the antibiotics my instinct told me she needed when I first bought her in! Even reading this, I am sure you will feel my despair at what my daughter had been through. I felt like I had been railroaded into treatments and my views ignored. Granted, I was not a trained medic, but I knew my daughter and her medical history better than anyone else, and my opinions should not have been disregarded. I knew then that I would have to learn to be a more vocal and knowledgeable advocate for my children in future. 'Experts' are still people, and people make mistakes. But when it comes to health, mistakes cost lives.

My daughter was immediately put on both intravenous and oral antibiotics to clear the infection but remained in the hospital for five days. Even after she was discharged, she had to be gradually weaned off the unnecessary salbutamol as it is a steroid medication, and abrupt withdrawal of the drug would cause nasty side effects. She was also placed under the care of a pediatric cardiologist because the salbutamol had caused her to develop a heart murmur that needed to be monitored. I was informed that her chest would be weak from now on and that she would likely need nebulizer treatment if she contracted any future influenza or viral infections. What total incompetent madness. I was so angry. There was no word of apology for the errors in her care. I felt like it was all just swept under the carpet. What was that all about? She went to the hospital with a chest infection but was almost killed by a little-known word called iatrogenesis.

Iatrogenesis comes from two Greek words; 'iatros', which means physician, and 'genesis', which means beginning or origin. Hence, iatrogenesis literally means conditions or ailments caused by physicians. It is the death or dangerous side effects of being treated by your doctor or physician. Unfortunately, these adverse effects are so common now that according to a study published by John Hopkins, it is currently the third largest cause of death in the United States, with almost 10%

of all deaths in the United States attributed to medical error. (33) Yet you will not see those figures reported in the newspapers. Furthermore, this figure is only a fraction of the problem as it only includes deaths but does not include patients damaged by their prescribed medications or those requiring other prescription medications to control the side effects (iatrogenesis) of the primary drug prescription.

The World Health Organization defines iatrogenesis as "any noxious, unintended, and undesired effect of a drug which occurs at doses used in humans (that means normal doses accepted as 'safe') for prophylaxis (prevention, e.g., vaccines), diagnosis, or therapy." (26)

Consider these statistics published in Duluth Reader in August 2019, from an article entitled "Is US Health Really the Best in The World?" It was written by Barbara Stanfield, MD, MPH, and published in the *Journal of the American Medical Association.* (32)

In the article, Stanfield included the following statistics from her research on America's iatrogenic deaths:

- 12,000 deaths/year from unnecessary surgery in hospitals
- 7,000 deaths/year from medication errors in hospitals
- 20,000 deaths/year from other errors in hospitals
- 80,000 deaths/year from nosocomial infections (meaning infections that were contracted whilst admitted as an inpatient in a hospital)
- *106,000 deaths/year from non-error, adverse effects of medications in hospitals* (italics mine to highlight this one)

Combining these five groups gives us a total of 225,000 inpatient deaths. The 225,000 number does not include out-patient iatrogenic deaths that occur at home, iatrogenic nursing home deaths or even non-lethal, chronic illnesses or disabilities. In any case, this number alone easily constitutes the third leading cause of death in the United States, behind heart disease and cancer. Even worse, these figures are only for the US. If we were to discover the global totals, they would be terrifying!

Note that Stanfield also did not present any data about iatrogenic drug- or vaccine-induced disorders that did NOT result in death. If there were such retrievable data, it could be reasonably asserted that iatrogenic disorders are the most common cause of acute or chronic/disabling diseases in the United States.

Despite its prevalence, I would not be surprised if you had never heard of iatrogenesis. It is often quietly swept under the carpet and hidden from public view, most likely to prevent the public outcry that would ensue if it became known. It was this that almost killed my young daughter; iatrogenesis, not asthma, not a chest infection, but the toxic effects of the treatments prescribed by her physicians because of their misdiagnosis. However, iatrogenesis is not always as dramatic as this and can often go slyly unnoticed as a result.

For example, eczema patients usually visit their doctor wondering what their or their child's rash could be. They are often diagnosed with eczema, generally with no further explanation other than being caused by excessively dry skin and commonly being an inherited condition. Having been 'diagnosed' with eczema, if we are lucky, we are taught the standard treatment protocol, which is to educate us in the concept of self-management, providing instructions on how to manage and replace moisture levels in the skin using petrochemical-based emollients and soap substitutes. Frequent use of these emollients, we are told, will help to restore the weak skin barrier, along with oil baths and topical application of moisturizers. We are also prescribed anti-inflammatory treatments, for example, topical steroids, with instructions to use them sparingly, only when eczema is particularly inflamed and raw, with a warning that they can cause thinning of the skin. This is true, but eczema patients are rarely told what the implications of this skin thinning are. Steroid creams suppress the immune function in the skin while also thinning the skin and allowing it to be penetrated more easily by irritants. This leads to dependencies developing and horrible withdrawal effects, which have only recently begun to receive recognition and have been given the labels topical steroid withdrawal, topical steroid withdrawal syndrome, or red skin syndrome. It can be life-changing and traumatizing due to the severity and duration it takes to recover skin health. (109) Topical steroids can also cause the pigment in the skin to be affected in people of colour. I believe they can contribute to the development of pityriasis alba, where the skin develops white patches of reduced pigment that resemble vitiligo. One of my daughters developed this. We were advised it was likely caused by repeated steroid use when she was younger. This is an example of the often-unnoticed episodes of iatrogenesis. Thankfully, it did resolve in time with proper skin care, but it is important to realize that iatrogenesis is not always immediately noticeable. The connection is often missed entirely because the insidious side effects of medical treatments can manifest many years later. An example of this is a little girl I met who was diagnosed with osteoporosis at only eight-years old after being prescribed oral steroids for two years to treat severe eczema.

Other protocols are prescribed as standard if eczema is not managed well by the measures previously mentioned. These can include calcineurin inhibitors, antiseptics, and wet wraps, to name a few. Ultraviolet long-wave treatments have helped some patients, and others have been prescribed topical antifungals and systemic antibiotics. (8, 16) Doxycycline is prescribed as a long-term antibiotic due to its effectiveness against *Staphylococcus* infection; however, it has been shown in studies to have a detrimental effect on the gut microbiome, and we now know a healthy microbiome is essential to our physical and mental health. We will cover more about the noxious results of this in a later chapter, but for now, be assured that wiping out your gut flora is not a desirable outcome and is another example of iatrogenesis that has far-reaching but not immediately noticeable effects. Doxycycline can also cause some rather nasty withdrawal effects, which can involve the skin, sinuses, and urinary tract if patients try to come off it without planning a slow tapered withdrawal. My clients are often on numerous medications to manage eczema and other health conditions and are shocked when I point out the known side effects of their medications. Many of these drugs list pruritus (skin itching), skin rashes, and dermatitis as known and common side effects. It is ridiculously counter-productive to be treating eczema patients with medications that cause eczema-like side effects. Do you not agree? In addition, it would be just as counter-productive for me not to point this out as I would be attempting to guide them to freedom while they are continuing to take substances that cause the iatrogenesis that is perpetuating the eczema.

An enlightened quote by Voltaire states, "Doctors are men who prescribe medications of which they know little, to cure diseases of which they know less, in people of whom they know nothing." When you look at "health care" through the lens of this quote, it is hardly surprising that iatrogenesis is so prevalent. Ensuring that people understand the side effects of any medication they are taking for ANY current health conditions is an essential aspect of working towards eczema healing. It should also be compulsory BEFORE prescribing them, as otherwise, there has been no genuinely informed consent. However, in our present climate of censorship and singular approved narratives, one must question whether even our doctors have access to complete, uncensored information on which to base their recommendations. Having said this, I DO NOT advocate suddenly withdrawing yourself from any medications. This can be extremely dangerous and should only be done under the care and supervision of your doctor. Again, I reiterate I am not a doctor. I educate and provide the resources for you to advocate for yourself and your loved ones. As eczema patients correct the root causes of their eczema, they can typically phase a gradual, safe withdrawal from their eczema medications without causing significant withdrawal symptoms. Additionally, they can work with their medical professionals to move to other non-conflicting medicines for any other health concerns. (Although as people correct the internal issues causing eczema, other health issues have also been seen to improve or resolve.)

Depending on the severity of the eczema rash you present to your physician, you may be prescribed antihistamines to help alleviate the itching. These are also prescribed to break the itch-scratch cycle and allow time for the skin to heal between flare-ups. This is often the case when atopic eczema is involved with the development of allergies. My children had 18 different food allergies between them and an additional four environmental allergies. None of them had all the same allergies, so you can imagine how interesting it was for me trying to prepare nutritional family meals. (Perhaps all my allergy-free recipes will be another book project in the future.) My son was even allergic to tap water, so bathing was forced to be a quick dip, soap, rinse, and out before he became covered in hives!

Allergies can exacerbate eczema symptoms, which was the case in my family. Consequently, additional antihistamines were prescribed in addition to the chlorphenamine we purchased at the pharmacy. The medication prescribed was not licensed for use in children under two years of age, and my daughter was only four months old. However, her consultant considered that she needed the intervention to reduce the itching and resultant scratching to allow her skin a respite period in which to recover. I was advised to keep her on this medication until she was two years old. However, I did not want any of my children to become dependent on long-term drugs. Therefore, as soon as her skin irritation was under control, I gradually weaned her off the medication, reducing the dose by imperceptible amounts every few days. By doing this, I did not cause any kick-back reactions from having a sudden increase in her histamine levels.

What is histamine? Histamine is a substance produced by cells during an allergic reaction and is one of the substances that causes the itching sensation in the skin. It is what causes the itchy bump to appear in a positive skin prick allergy test. Antihistamines are, as the name suggests, histamine antagonists, meaning they block the action of histamine. In theory, it sounds like a great idea to take them regularly, but when you do not know how to heal internally, the intervention becomes a long-term dependency instead of short-term symptomatic relief. In addition, with long-term antihistamine use having been associated with the iatrogenic development of neurological problems in later life, you want to avoid complacently staying on them if there is a better way.

Medicines can also lose effectiveness over extended periods because they operate like a gag to stop the body from shouting at you that

---

something is wrong. Your body is shouting because it needs your help to correct an issue. Let me reiterate what I said earlier; if you ignore its cries or try to suppress it, it will start to shout even louder at you. It could be in the form of the drugs ceasing to work, although it is often through the development of new and additional symptoms. You are then faced with a choice, take even stronger pharmaceutical gags or start to listen to your body and find out how to help it.

When other interventions have failed or lost effectiveness over time, immune suppressant drugs and oral steroids can be prescribed instead. Unfortunately, these come not only with a hefty price tag (if you do not have health insurance or a subsidized National Health Service) but also a hefty burden of side effects on the body. (16) As I mentioned previously, I have personally seen an 8-year-old develop osteoporosis from long-term oral steroid use to control severe eczema. In addition, I have witnessed adults develop cancer after taking immune suppressants for autoimmune diseases. This iatrogenesis should be classed as medical malpractice, as the Hippocratic oath of medical professionals includes "Do no harm." I believe no one should be put on medication with such potentially toxic side effects, least of all children, unless for life-saving intervention or to provide relief from debilitating symptoms **whilst investigating the root cause**. Dupixent is now approved for use in children as young as six, and the Federal Drug Administration also approved immune suppressants called JAK inhibitors. However, I feel we are on a dangerous path as we have not been using these drugs for long enough to have ascertained the long-term risks associated with making 'adjustments' to our intricate immune systems, especially those of developing children. Instead, I believe the goal should always be to identify the problem, address it, and then gradually withdraw the medication as safely as possible as the cause is resolved.

Despite all these treatment options and the copious expenditure on research, people have yet to investigate why some treatments work for some people but not others, nor why some people develop worsened conditions by treatments that appear to help others. There are many variables, such as our genetics and microbiome condition, that directly alter how our body responds to pharmaceutical drugs. Unless you have the funds to pay for private testing to check your genetic makeup and microbiome to assess your likely response to drugs, trying to manage disease symptoms with medications can be like playing a game of Russian Roulette, where you do not know whether the chamber is loaded against you or not. Similarly, without investigation, the treatment of eczema can become like a doctor's pick-and-mix chocolate box with a missing contents leaflet, where they try to pick the best option from a choice of colourful wrappers without really knowing the end result. I am not saying that we should never use medications as they have saved countless lives when used in emergencies and provided much relief to suffering people. However, we should not live our lives dependent upon them. Instead, we should make every effort to investigate and treat the root cause of our disease.

The internet is awash with alternate therapies. Amid so much conflicting advice though, it is often easier to go with the status quo and follow the instructions of your medical practitioner, even though it is not working, especially if you feel worn down by all the disappointments you have experienced in your eczema journey. In addition, we have been conditioned to follow medical advice and not to question those in authority who obviously know better than us by virtue of their medical training, just as I did when my daughter was in the hospital. However, it eventually becomes apparent, even to the most die-hard pharmaceutical advocates, that these protocols barely manage the symptoms of eczema and are certainly not providing long-term healing.

There are also other burdens to consider. Eczema rashes are intensely itchy, and trying not to scratch is extremely challenging, especially at night. In particular, children claw at their skin while they sleep and can also be most ingenious at extricating themselves from the various eczema clothing barriers we parents use to stop the scratching. My kids certainly were. They constantly scratched and rubbed the itching areas in a vain attempt to alleviate the irritation. I lost count of how many times I put them to bed believing their hands were effectively covered with eczema clothing solutions and their little faces safe from clawing fingernails, only to find my escapologists had extricated themselves and slashed their faces despite my attempts to keep their fingernails as short as possible and their hands covered.

The burden of disrupted sleep affects both adult and child eczema patients along with their parents or spouses. How many hours of productive work are lost because people are just so exhausted from negotiating eczema at night when all they want is a good night's sleep after an equally exhausting day trying to deal with it?

I also dread to think how much money I spent on various eczema 'solutions' over the years. All these products and medications cost money, particularly when we are left to try an endless array of products in our attempts to find something that remotely works at all. I found it interesting that patients with eczema and allergies can be classed as disabled in the United States if it significantly affects their ability to function in life. In the United Kingdom, there is no such classification; however, I would have greatly appreciated the help of a disability allowance to offset some of the costs of allergy-free foods, creams, supplements, and eczema clothing, especially as I stopped working to care for my four eczematous and allergic children. Eczema costs money and creates a financial burden on the sufferer and their family. Such costs include eczema clothing, alternative bedding, dust mite covers, emollient creams, and prescription costs. These are in addition to the cost of allergy-free foods to negotiate the 'Allergic March' that invariably develops and the cost of lost income when adults either leave work to care for younger sufferers as I did or find they do not achieve the sales results or promotions at work because they are judged on the appearance of their skin, not their abilities.

Insurance companies and the National Health Service in the United Kingdom are carrying an ever-increasing burden to fund the long-term medications prescribed in attempts to alleviate this condition. Yet despite the financial outlay, it is still considered an 'incurable' disease, with all those medications being only a means of symptom management (and a great source of revenue for the pharmaceutical industry).

We can feel heartbroken at our children's broken and bleeding skin, yet even worse problems occur when it continues over an extended period. That constant pressure on the skin of clawing, rubbing, and scratching, can lead to a thickening of the skin over time, which causes it to take on the appearance of leather. This is known as lichenification. The word comes from a root, which literally means 'turning to leather'. It occurs because the cells in the epidermis (the upper skin layer) grow more rapidly in response to the friction of rubbing and itching. However, when it occurs too often, the epidermis will start to produce cells faster despite the shedding from the upper layer occurring at the same rate as before. This allows the body to build up a thicker skin layer as a form of protection, almost like a callous, enabling it to better withstand the pressures it is being subjected to. (27) This is one of the reasons why allowing children to scratch until they bleed is highly detrimental, contrary to what some alternative eczema healers promote. Allowing this will cause unattractive lichenification and scarring, which at the very least causes self-consciousness and embarrassment (yet another emotional and physical burden), and, at worst, can lead to life-threatening bacterial infections. Please do not allow your children to scratch until they bleed. It does not release toxins from the body, as some people state, but it does increase the likelihood of bacterial invasions, a hyperactive immune response, and scarring. There are far more helpful ways to reduce itching that do not risk harm; a cold compress is the simplest and easiest to implement. Cooling the inflamed patch reduces blood flow to the area and consequently reduces the immune response causing the itching. I will cover the mechanisms of this in a later chapter. In the meantime, cold compresses should be your first point of call for any patches of eczema that make you or your child feel like you want to claw your skin off. In the case of children, having cooling packs readily available when they are needed also allows them to feel more in control of managing their eczema. If you use ice packs, ensure you wrap a cloth around the packs to avoid any ice burns on the skin. Cold, not freezing, is optimal.

The physical manifestations of eczema also bring emotional and psychological burdens to bear. For example, a child's most formative years for learning to bond and receive affection are from the ages of 0-3 years, when every hug, tickle, and baby massage causes neuronal connections to form in the brain. Yet with moderate-to-severe eczema, the infant often cannot bear to receive these types of physical affection because of the discomfort it causes them. One of my daughters was so covered in eczema that she could not bear to be held. Anything that made her feel hot was too uncomfortable for her, whether that was a cuddle or the car safety seat. Car journeys were often a nightmare, as it would not have been safe to travel without her being in the car seat, yet she would often cry and fight the whole journey while strapped in there. Sadly, these babies are denied, through no fault of their own, much of life's everyday comforts or relational affection simply because it causes them so much discomfort. As a direct result of the torment of living with endless itching that seems to show no sign of mercy, these children live with excessive and abnormal stress levels, which can cause lasting emotional, physiological, and relational impacts. If it persists into adulthood, statistics show that adults suffering from chronic eczema also live with elevated levels of stress due to negotiating a chronic illness, which affects their work, sleep, and social acceptance. Sadly, people with eczema have a higher rate of suicide than those who do not. One only needs to read the frequent posts in eczema support forums and Facebook groups to see the repeatedly asked questions begging for ideas to find relief from torment. The questions provide a sad insight into the frustration and desperation of eczema patients longing to find freedom from either their own or their children's suffering. Many years ago, I was one of them, googling and searching the internet intently, trying to understand what I could do to help my precious babies. It saddens me that although there are so many questions, unfortunately, there are also as many conflicting answers, resulting in more confusion rather than help.

A further issue to be aware of is that eczema patients also bear a higher burden of autoimmune diseases than non-eczema patients. This is because they experience detrimental chronic adaptions in the immune and stress response and even in gene expression (in which gene 'switches' are turned on and off). Many other conditions are significantly related to eczema, but most people are unaware that chronic eczema causes internal changes that make them susceptible to developing these conditions. Studies have shown that children with eczema have double the risk of developing all types of autoimmune diseases and that adult eczema patients also have a vastly increased risk of developing autoimmune diseases. Conditions such as asthma, allergies, hay fever, psoriasis, alopecia, urticaria, Sjogren syndrome, lupus, Crohn's disease, celiac disease, irritable bowel syndrome, ankylosing spondylitis, rheumatoid arthritis, and depression, to name a few, are common amongst eczema patients. (31) This is because the body of an eczema patient is continuing to cry out for help, but it is being ignored as people simply do not know what to do. However, when the root problem is not addressed, it will continue to spread, just like bad fruit on the diseased tree. Furthermore, the very fact that it IS so common for the diseased fruit to spread leads medics to EXPECT the development of additional diseases, just as they expected asthma with my daughter. The doctors assumed an asthma attack because it is considered 'normal' for eczema patients to develop allergies and asthma. This is known as atopic disease or the 'Allergic March'. However, it is now my opinion that the allergic march is simply another mechanism for the body to cry more loudly to get our attention.

Although eczema is recognized as afflicting more young children and that they will hopefully 'grow out of it', it can also occur for the first time later in life, or if unresolved, it can remain into adult life. After resolving the eczema present in my children, I developed it myself for the first time in my forties. However, I knew why it had occurred after referring to my Eczemology™ Map and was able to heal myself very quickly. I will share that story with you later.

There are currently millions of adults around the world living with this awful condition. At the time of writing this book, the current estimates are over 230 million eczema sufferers worldwide. (36) It is said to affect up to 20% of children and 3% of adults globally. (8) No, you are not alone in your suffering.

As our understanding of eczema evolves, it is becoming apparent that its burdens extend far beyond the boundaries that we defined for it. Although eczema has traditionally been considered a skin disorder or dermatology issue, it is neither limited to that domain in its cause nor does it remain there in its effects. More recently, research has revealed that eczema has many internal complexities, even from its origin. Scientific papers now report that immune dysfunction is involved, along with gut issues, toxic overload, gene mutations, and more. Therefore, simply advising people to slather on various emollients multiple times a day is clearly leaving patients devoid of adequate care and education. It instead leaves them to shoulder a heavy burden that is entirely unnecessary.

I have made my point. Eczema causes burdens that far exceed the boundaries we have set for it, and we urgently need to escape its clutches.

If you have been let down many times, you may be feeling frustrated or hopeless. I frequently hear eczema sufferers say defeated words like "I do not think there is any hope for me" or "I have already tried everything." You may genuinely feel like this, but let me tell you, it is not true. We can all be guilty of exaggerating, and it is usually because we are building a wall to protect ourselves from further hurt and disappointment. The truth is that you have NOT tried everything. I guarantee you have not tried the things I will teach you in this book, which have been proven, by the researchers involved, to get results. We create a powerful synergistic solution when we combine them and bring these protocols from many different angles simultaneously. So, whenever you catch yourself thinking that this probably will not work for you, recognize it for what it is – a misplaced self-sabotage mechanism trying to protect you from perceived failure (again). Instead of focusing on your fears, focus on what your ideal result would look like.

What would your perfect day be? A day with no itching at all? Or being able to function normally throughout the day without worrying about somehow triggering a flare-up? Is it confidently stepping outside in shorts and a t-shirt, knowing that your skin is clear, with no concerns about how people will look at you? Is it being able to focus on your work without being embarrassed by the flakes of dry skin covering your desk, or is it sleeping peacefully and comfortably through the night? Whatever you desire is possible, but you must start focusing on where you want to go, not what failed in the past or what you are afraid of. Yes, you may have been disappointed before. I went through a lot of disappointment before discovering these answers. I totally understand how you feel. But now you can learn from me. I have built a bridge to get you from where you are now to where you want to be without you having to do all the research yourself. Remember, you can never drive forward if you insist on looking only in the rearview mirror. Healing is possible. Please remember that if you need additional support, you can always contact me for personal coaching or to find out about my next course availability. I am here to help you. Let us look at the first eczema spider leg and determine what is going wrong with your skin.

SPIDER LEGS MAKE SPIDER WEBS

4

The Riddle of the Root

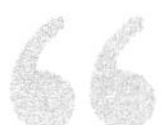 *Even with a newly diagnosed infant eczema, the roots can be traced back to before the child was born or even conceived."*

Even though I was only four years old, the Great Drought of 1976 must have had a significant impact on me because I can clearly remember some of the ramifications. That year, summer in the United Kingdom was blazing hot, with long, drawn sunny days and uncomfortable sticky nights. The temperatures exceeded 38°C for the first time, with a new record set in Faversham, Kent. In a country that usually has summer heat for only two months of the year, we basked in five months of sunshine. Crowds fled the towns and flocked to the beaches seeking the cooling sea breezes. At first, it was wonderful, but a huge problem was brewing that most residents were blissfully unaware of at the beginning. The water supplies in the country were running seriously low.

The drought did not suddenly occur as a single event in 1976. The roots of the drought were laid during the previous 5-year period, which had been the driest on record since the 1850s. This was followed by the driest period since records began back in 1717, lasting from May 1975 to August 1976. Even the winter season of 1975 yielded little water, neither as rain nor snow. Consequently, as the spring of 1976 arrived, reservoirs in the United Kingdom were barely at half their normal capacity, and the groundwater had already been diminished. The heatwave then began, and demand for water increased; there were thirsty people, thirsty farm animals, and parched crops. Water restrictions were put in place as the heatwave and drought continued. By July, the situation had become so severe that drastic measures were taken to shut off the water supplies to residential houses. Standpipes were installed in communities where families would come and collect their water ration for the day. There was one standpipe for every 20 homes. This is one of the things I remember clearly, standing at the end of our road, queuing in a long line with our neighbours to collect our daily water supply. The drought and heatwave showed no sign of abating, and in early August 1976, London had only 90 days of water supply left in its reservoirs. You may be wondering why I am telling you all about the Great United Kingdom Drought, but please bear with me as it correlates to the development of eczema.

The drought had many wider ramifications. According to a historical article about the Great Drought of 1976, published in Countryfile Magazine, the heat was so intense that tarmac roads melted and remained viscous, fish perished in their thousands as the rivers and lakes dried up, and masses of birds died from botulism as the only water they could find was stagnant and disease-ridden. Farms also struggled as crop harvests failed from the lack of water. The United Kingdom became a place of forest fires and burning heaths, with over half of Surrey Heath being destroyed by fire, in addition to the destruction caused to heathland elsewhere in the country. Furthermore, over 2000 hectares of forestlands were destroyed. As the water supply situation was critical, many heath fires were left to burn unabated apart from fire breaks. There simply was not enough water left for the fire brigade to use on the fires. In addition to this devastation, thousands of native Elm trees were killed by an outbreak of Dutch Elm disease after being weakened by the drought conditions and subsequently attacked by an overpopulation of Vector Beetles. Next came invasions of green flies and aphids, which caused the ladybird population to burgeon to almost plague-like proportions due to the abundance of aphid food. However, as the aphid and green fly populations diminished, the hungry ladybirds started to bite humans instead. There were reports of people running from beaches to escape ladybird swarms, farming machines being jammed up by huge ladybird colonies, and light aircraft disappearing amidst swarms of these flying bugs.

I also remember the state of the ground, possibly because I was closer to it than most being so small; I was fascinated by the cracked patterns appearing in the soil. The water had long evaporated, and with the ferocious sun baking the clay soil relentlessly day after day, everywhere was parched and cracked open in a myriad of abstract shapes to pique my young imagination. The topsoil became powdery dust that blew away in swirls and whirls. At our local secondary school, the cracks in the front grounds were so large they looked like chasms in my four-year-old eyes. I remember hearing my parents talking about a small first former who had fallen right down into one of the cracks and had to be pulled out.

The following picture looks like the ground during the summer of 1976. It also resembles eczema skin, which is going through its own type of drought; it is parched and cracked. Water is evaporating faster than it can be replaced, and irritants are slipping through the cracks. But why is this happening? What is causing this rapid water loss and cracking? Just as the drought of 1976 had roots that began many years earlier, in a similar fashion, eczema also has roots that span back many years too. Yes, even with a newly diagnosed infant, the roots can be traced back to before the child was born or even conceived.

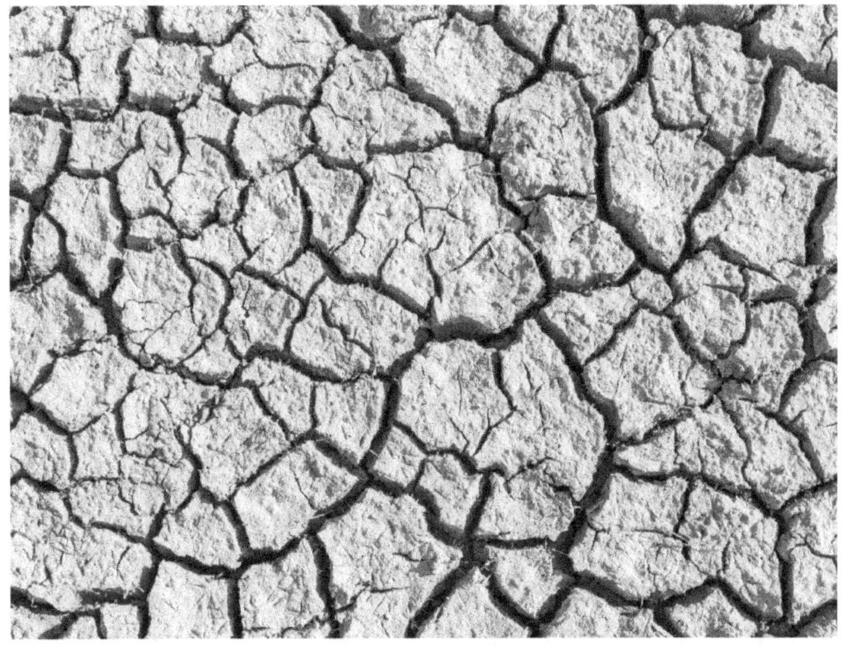

Genetic susceptibility and unresolved 'droughts' in the maternal mothers' life certainly load the gun in favour of eczema development, but there is usually a subsequent event that pulls the trigger.

In this section of the book, we will start peeling back the layers of the onion and looking a little deeper each time until we reveal the Riddle of the Root. Let us first look at how eczema typically develops.

If we look at the pattern of eczema in children, it typically follows a well-known progression path. It commonly begins with cradle cap in infants at around 8-12 weeks old and the development of excessively dry skin. However, even though this is often not recognized as an early sign of eczema, it shows that the skin's natural moisturizing factor (NMF) is not performing optimally, and there is a lack of sebum protecting the skin. There is a short window here where if this red flag is heeded and corrective interventions are taken, I believe eczema can be avoided altogether. Sadly though, the development of cradle cap is most often overlooked, or parents are just told to use specific shampoos or to rub oil into the scalp to loosen the skin scales. Consequently, with root causes left untreated, the eczema rash typically develops on the face, usually the cheeks, at around eight weeks of age, followed by the flexor regions of arms and legs (the folding areas inside the elbows and behind the knees). Later, the usual pattern of eczema is a spread to the neck creases, where sweat accumulates, then to the hands, and in severe cases, it can spread widely and affect large areas of the body. This happened with my second daughter. Eczema also tends to be accompanied by generally dry skin over much of the body. (One of my daughters had skin so dry it felt like fragile tissue paper.) This is said to occur because of excessive water loss from both the dermal (lower) and epidermal (upper) layers of skin (much like the excessive water loss from the clay soil in the Great Drought) (16) but without explaining WHY there is excessive water loss. However, eczema does not always follow this typical pattern. Some children are born with extremely dry skin, and some develop eczema in their teens. Similarly, adults can suddenly be afflicted with eczema in later life and are often perplexed as to why? When eczema first occurs is an important clue in solving the 'Riddle of the Root'.

I mentioned earlier the loss of an effective natural moisturizing barrier and the lack of sebum. These are both essential to maintain correct skin hydration levels of water and lipids (natural oils). A deficiency in either or both will result in a substandard skin barrier function as they not only keep moisture in but also assist in keeping other substances out. Consequently, this defective barrier allows excess water loss via evaporation from your skin layers. Although emollients are typically prescribed to attempt to replenish the moisture levels, the underlying causes still need to be addressed. Furthermore, even the best emollients in the world are a poor substitute for a perfectly suited, naturally formed natural moisturizing factor. I will talk more about the natural moisturizing factor shortly.

My first port of call in identifying what went wrong inside my children was to look at eczematous skin compared to healthy skin. That is when I learned how amazing the skin is.

I remember growing up thinking that the skin only had one job, to hold everything inside my body, much like cling wrap holding produce inside supermarket packaging. I now know that our skin is incredible. Every square inch of skin has 20 blood vessels, 650 sweat glands, 1000 nerve endings, 60 thousand melanocytes (your skin colour or pigment-producing cells), and 19 million skin cells. We shed 30-40 thousand old skin cells every day, (25) the majority of which contributes to the dust we clean from our houses.

The skin helps to regulate our body temperature. It also houses our hair follicles, those minuscule factories that produce our hair and sebum. Healthy skin is covered in friendly microbes that help our immune system function effectively, protecting against pathogenic bacteria and toxic substances. Skin produces natural moisturizing factors and holds our nerve endings close to the surface, allowing us to sense if something is hot, cold, rough, smooth, or the sensation of pain. It also provides a fascinating window for revealing problems within the body. For example, if your skin turns yellow, it indicates a liver problem and too much bile in the bloodstream. If your skin becomes much paler than usual, it can indicate anaemia. Furthermore, if it turns blue, it indicates hypoxia or a lack of oxygen reaching the body tissues. This is common knowledge to doctors, yet they rarely ask what the appearance of eczema tells us.

Skin is the largest organ in the body, weighing in at between 7.5 and 22 lbs. (depending on a person's body size), with a surface area of 1.5 to 2 m^2. We often fail to realize the significance of our skin being this large. By virtue of its size, it plays an incredibly active role in detoxifying the body, especially if the other waste processing systems are overloaded or functioning less optimally. Skin can degrade, inactivate, and eliminate numerous synthetic chemicals that are foreign to our body's ecological system (called xenobiotics) and other toxins that originate from within us as a natural byproduct of our existence (called endogenous toxic compounds). It does this through a variety of mechanisms, including xenobiotic and drug-metabolizing enzymes, the reactive oxygen species-scavenging system (a form of antioxidant), and sweat glands, which eliminate toxins and water-soluble crystals such as uric acid from the body in the form of sweat. (28) When the skin is healthy and functioning optimally, it does a fantastic job of helping us to detoxify. However, when, for various reasons, it is not able to function correctly, it cannot aid the detoxifying processes, and those waste products begin to build up inside us. This is even more pronounced when the microbiome is imbalanced too. I will explain this in detail in a later chapter.

Skin is one of those many precious things that we take for granted until something goes wrong. It is responsible for so much more than just holding our body together, yet too often, we do not give it much thought until problems develop. We may exhibit skin issues that last for a short time, like a viral rash or a reaction to something in our environment. Puberty can arrive with its flight-case of skin problems like acne and boils, or as we advance in years, we may notice the development of wrinkles and sagging skin. Menopause can cause the skin to become excessively dry because of hormonal fluctuations. All these can be prompts that cause us to seek better skincare and realize we cannot take it for granted. However, with chronic conditions, such as eczema, our thoughts about skin can go from virtually nonexistent to an almost obsessive barrage of endless questions and searching for answers.

The first step on the road to recovery is to understand how healthy skin should form. Once we have laid that foundation, we can compare eczematous skin and look at what has gone wrong. Although this section does get a little technical, please do not skip it. It really is extremely helpful to grasp this, as in later chapters, I refer to the teaching on the structure of the skin to show how the strands of the web feed into each other and perpetuate the eczema state. I promise not to make it too overbearing.

Look at the picture below. You will see that skin has two main sections or layers. The dermis is the deeper skin layer, and the epidermis is the upper layer – the skin you can see. The dermis is much thicker than the epidermis. It consists of tough connective tissue, which houses your blood vessels, nerve endings, hair follicles, and sweat glands. The blood vessels in the dermis are essential as they not only carry oxygen and nutrients right up to the lower layer of the epidermis but immune cells too. The actions of the immune cells are primarily responsible for the inflammation that occurs in eczematous skin; we will look at the inflammatory cycles in a subsequent chapter.

Skin Anatomy

The subcutaneous tissue is the layer of fat at the bottom, which provides a layer of insulation, amongst other things.

Sebaceous glands in the dermis produce a substance called sebum, which is vital to healthy skin. It is an oily substance that is secreted into the hair follicles and makes its way to the skin's surface, providing a waterproof coating to both hair and skin. This coating helps to prevent them from drying out. Sebum also has important antibacterial properties that inhibit the growth of unwanted micro-organisms in the skin, such as pathogenic bacteria and fungi. Eczematous skin typically has less sebum than healthy skin and consequently reduced antibacterial protection, which contributes to the increased colonization of pathogenic micro-organisms in comparison to healthy skin. Eczema patients are typically told that their skin lacks sufficient sebum, which is often the only explanation given for having eczema, apart from the flippant "It is genetic." Emollients are commonly prescribed to plug the moisture gap. However, while insufficient sebum is predominantly true, it is only a tiny portion of the complex equation. Slathering on emollients does nothing to replace the antibacterial properties that are deficient. In addition, if we use antibacterial emollients, they indiscriminately kill all the micro-organisms on the skin, including the ones that are beneficial to us, which causes further problems.

Various cells reside in the dermis, including mast cells, vascular smooth muscle cells, specialized muscle cells, fibroblasts, and immune cells. They all have distinct roles to play.

Mast cells are like sentry guardsmen. They stand on guard around all the perimeter fences of your body, such as under your skin. Mast cells are responsible for dumping granular mediators into the skin when they are disturbed. It is these granules that cause hives, rashes, and itching during allergic reactions in addition to vasoconstriction (tightening of blood vessels) and bronchoconstriction (narrowing of the airways) seen in severe reactions and allergic asthma. Understanding the action of mast cells is especially important in overcoming eczema because they are directly involved in one of the loop systems we need to switch off. When I teach about the immune and allergy cycles, I use the cartoon characters of the immune cells from my **Superheroes Inside Me** book, making it much easier to follow.

The vascular smooth muscle cells allow blood vessels to contract and dilate, regulating body temperature. Dilation of blood vessels increases blood flow to the upper levels, and contracting them decreases blood flow near the skin's surface.

When the body is hot, increasing blood flow near the surface allows heat to be lost through the skin. In contrast, when the body is too cold, the flow will be decreased to reduce heat loss and protect the internal organs from the cold, as the blood flow will be more directed to these vital organs. This explains why cold compresses work to reduce itching. Applying cold has the effect of contracting the blood vessels and reducing the flow of blood to the area. Consequently, the number of immune cells migrating to the site also decreases; thus, the inflammatory response is reduced.

Vascular smooth muscle cells also cause blood vessels to dilate in response to messages received from your immune system regarding invasion, injury, or infection. Dilation increases blood flow to the area and consequently allows the influx of other immune cells to assist during episodes of inflammation or injury. This partly explains why eczema sufferers often say strenuous exercise exacerbates itching and flares. As the vascular smooth muscle cells dilate to allow more blood to flow to the surface for heat evaporation, it has the unfortunate side effect of bringing more immune cells to the surface to identify and respond to the irritation or breeches in the skin barrier, which then triggers a greater inflammatory response. I will address exercise in more detail later.

Specialized muscle cells, found around the sweat glands, contract to expel the sweat out of our sweat glands, helping us to reduce body heat via sweat evaporation when we are too hot. We can also expel toxins through our sweat too, so regular exercise that works up a little sweat is a good thing to help our bodies detoxify. However, the trick is to balance your exercise; this should be enough to give strength, respiratory, and detoxification benefits without pushing yourself so hard that you suppress your innate immune system or overheat and inadvertently bring an influx of immune cells to the surface of the skin. The salt and slight acidity of your sweat can also irritate areas of skin affected by eczema. Sweat that has been blocked from evaporating by petroleum-based emollients can also build up under the skin and then leach into the surrounding tissues. This can cause an immune response, which subsequently leads to the development of an allergy to your own sweat and is another reason why sweating can exacerbate eczema. Thus, avoiding petroleum-based emollients, using a fan or air conditioning whilst exercising, and showering quickly afterwards can all help mitigate these reactions.

Fibroblasts are cells that like that act like builders. They have a maintenance role in the body, a bit like caretakers, helping with repairs. They deposit collagen and other elements of the dermis layer as required for growth or to repair wounds and are also involved in the growth and maintenance of our bones. Fibroblasts can change roles to fibroclasts, which act as cleaners rather than builders, when there is debris and damaged tissues to clear out, perhaps from an injury or previous inflammation. We need fibroblasts to be healthy and robust as they are involved in repairing the damage to the skin because of eczema.

Then there are many variations of immune cells, including macrophages, which engulf and 'eat' foreign, degraded, or dead material. The name macrophage can literally be translated to 'big eater'. It is the perfect name for them as they eat invaders and degraded material in your body. Honestly, the immune system is so complex and intricate; it is like you have a whole universe of species inside your body. All the different types of cells have various jobs. When everything works in synergy, as it is designed to do, the harmony and genius of the system are utterly amazing. It reminds me of a nation's armed forces, with many players in various divisions, all working together and collaborating to achieve a common goal.

Many of your immune cells produce cytokine 'messengers' that have a variety of roles. For example, some 'recruit' other immune players to drive the inflammatory response during viral or bacterial invasions or after an injury, and some reduce it after the problem resolves. Cytokines play many different roles, and we will delve into these in Chapter 7, as some are particularly pertinent to eczema and are involved in the inflammatory cycles that drive flare-ups.

Your immune cells do not reside permanently in the skin; they exit the blood through the blood vessel wall and migrate into the skin layers to help destroy infections and invading bacteria when they are summoned by cytokines. In addition, they can travel to the lymph system to recruit other immune reinforcements when needed. These include the following cell types.

Neutrophils. These are usually the fastest responders to arrive at the site of inflammation. They also destroy invaders.

Dendritic cells. These are part of the same group as macrophages and neutrophils. They are white blood cells known as phagocytes, as they destroy invaders through a process called phagocytosis, which is essentially eating and digesting them.

T and B cells. These are also immune cells. They arrive more slowly but work together in the crucial role of making antibodies to viruses and bacteria. Once this task is performed, many of the mature B cells become memory cells, which hang around for a much longer time to provide faster responses in future 'invasions' of the same type. Memory B-cells are said to 'learn' to fight the diseases in previous infections or vaccines and then remain for long periods to provide antibody protection against further exposure to those diseases.

Eosinophils. These are specialized immune cells. They defend against parasitic and bacterial infections that have managed to break into our cells rather than those found in our fluids. They also modulate immediate allergic responses, such as allergic asthma and allergic skin responses. They do this by inactivating or cancelling the allergic mediators or substances released by the mast cells when they are disturbed, including chemicals such as histamine, leukotrienes, lysophospholipids, and heparin that typically cause irritation and itching. People who suffer from eczema and allergies tend to show more significant numbers of eosinophils in their blood than those who do not. The more allergies a person suffers, the greater the number of circulating eosinophils in their blood. This is because their efforts are constantly needed to restore equilibrium and mop up the allergic mediators released after exposure to allergens. (30)

If you are interested in learning more about the immune cells and how you can help them in their roles of looking after you, please consider checking out my previous book, **Superheroes Inside Me**, which is available on Amazon in both paperback and Kindle e-book versions. In this book, I turned the immune cells into Superheroes to teach people what they do through engaging and easy-to-understand stories and how our diet and lifestyle can affect their ability to protect us. You can find the Amazon link via my website or subscribe to read the first chapter for free.

https://www.superheroesinsideme.com

The upper layer of skin is called the epidermis. This is the layer I will focus more on examining, as it is where the major breakdowns occur in eczema. The epidermis is attached to the dermis by collagen fibres. These are the same collagen fibres that degenerate as we age, and as a result, our skin loses its elasticity and firmness, causing wrinkles and sagging skin. You have probably heard of collagen, as it is frequently added to skin care products, especially those in anti-ageing collections.

The epidermis contains melanocytes, which are the cells responsible for producing melanin. Melanin is produced when the skin is exposed to ultraviolet light and helps to protect it from damage. This is why people living in tropical climates close to the equator historically developed a darker skin colour to protect their skin from the intense ultraviolet rays of the sun. In contrast, those living far from the equator, with limited ultraviolet light exposure, developed pale skin. Exposure to ultraviolet light also causes the skin to produce vitamin D3 from cholesterol. However, vitamin D is not really a vitamin in the true sense. It is more like a hormone and is necessary for a vast number of processes in the body, including the correct working of transcription inside your cells (the copying and reading of your DNA instructions). It also affects how specific specialized cells differentiate, including keratinocyte skin cells, which are extremely important to our study. Having lighter skin enables those in areas of limited sunlight to produce vitamin D more efficiently, which is an adaptation that is essential to avoid deficiency. With many people emigrating to different continents nowadays, darker-skinned people who move to northern or southern climates have an elevated risk of developing high cholesterol as the ultraviolet rays are not strong enough to convert cholesterol to vitamin D3 as effectively in darker skin. In addition, they have a much higher risk of vitamin D deficiency resulting in more severe respiratory distress from viral infections and an increased risk of developing an impaired skin barrier function. It also increases the odds of developing many other diseases. Suffice to say, I always recommend that clients get their vitamin D levels checked and, if necessary, work with their medical advisor to increase the levels through supplementation until they are in the therapeutic range.

The epidermis is itself divided into layers. Most of the body has four layers of skin, and there is an additional fifth layer on the fingertips, soles of the feet, and palms of the hands. I concentrate on the four main layers in this book. However, if you suffer from eczema on your palms or the soles of your feet, the information here is still relevant, as the skin issues relating to eczema occur in these layers.

Look at the picture of the epidermis layers. I do not show all the layers of cells in this picture to save space.

Epidermis Layers

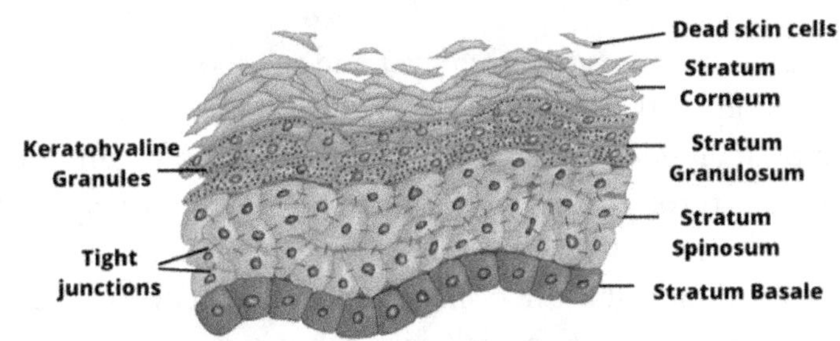

To explain what has gone wrong with your skin, I first need to show how your skin should form. So let me introduce you to the various skin layers in your epidermis and to expound on what each one does. I can then show you what is breaking down in your skin when you suffer from eczema.

The bottom layer is called the stratum basale. This layer of the epidermis is closest to the blood supply in the dermis and is only a single cell layer thick, around 0.025 millimetres! The stratum basale, the lower layer of the epidermis, is where your skin makes millions of new cells called keratinocytes every day; it is the only layer of your skin where your cells can divide and reproduce by mitosis (cell division). Yes, these are the same keratinocytes that require sufficient vitamin D to differentiate correctly, which makes it especially important for eczema patients to check their vitamin D status. Vitamin D deficiency can detrimentally affect the production of keratinocytes right at the offset of skin production.

The name keratinocyte comes from the word keratin. Keratin is a hard-structural protein. Its presence gives strength to our skin, hair, and nails. It will be a familiar word to anyone who reads their hair product labels, as it is commonly added as an ingredient to many products to increase hair strength. Keratinocytes are filled with keratin and carry it to the skin's surface, hence their name. Each day, as millions of new keratinocytes are made, this constant turnover pushes the previously made cells higher up the layers of skin. As we age, the production of new skin cells starts to decline. The cells gradually move up into the subsequent layers, where they continue to fill with keratin fibres and change their shape and composition.

The stratum spinosum is the next layer and sits above the stratum basale. It is around 8-10 cells thick. The cells continue to fill with keratin in this layer. If all goes well, the cells should take on a spiny shape as they move up through this layer of skin. The spines help them to interlock with each other, which provides extra strength to the layer of skin by forming tight junctions between cells. The picture shows spines between the cells. If you ball your hands into loose fists and push your knuckles together to interlock, that is similar to what your skin cells should do in the stratum spinosum. To produce these tight junctions, the skin must have enough of a protein called claudin 1. A study published in 2011 assessed the skin of eczema patients and found that they commonly show a deficiency of claudin 1. As a result, they do not produce the spiny tight junctions effectively. (29) In normal skin, claudin 1 proteins function as gates, playing an essential role in regulating the permeability of the epidermis (especially how much water can leave by evaporation and how easy it is for substances to enter the skin) and controlling the flow of substances inside the cells, such as hormones, cytokines, and electrolytes. (39) Therefore, a deficiency in claudin-1 protein will severely hamper the ability of the body to produce a healthy skin barrier. Without claudin-1, the junctions are ineffective; spaces develop between the cells, too much water evaporates out of the skin, and irritants can ingress more easily.

This is very similar to the ground in the Great Drought of 1976, which lost water faster than it could be replaced. As the water continued to evaporate from the ground, the soil became progressively drier until cracks appeared. The breaks and cracks allowed seeds to fall inside and take root (or small first formers to need rescuing). Without the claudin-1 proteins forming the tight junctions, skin becomes like the ground in a drought with too much water evaporating from the skin, leaving it to become excessively dry and crack open, allowing irritants and bacteria to invade below the surface.

As the keratinocyte cells continue to move further up, they enter the third layer, which is 3-5 cells thick, called the stratum granulosum, so named because the cells now contain granules called keratohyalin. These granules of keratin should now contain other proteins called histidine and cysteine. Histidine binds to water and effectively carries it in the cells to the upper layers of the skin, keeping it moist. It is then rapidly incorporated into a protein called profillagrin. Histidine and cysteine appear to bind the keratin filaments together, making them stronger. Histidine also has a role in regulating histamine release in the skin; histamine is involved in the allergic response, hence why we use antihistamines to alleviate allergic symptoms. Researchers have

identified that eczema skin has lower levels of histidine than non-
-eczema skin, which means that their skin cells are less efficient at holding and transporting water up through the skin layers, leaving their skin
dryer than normal. If you also have a deficiency in claudin 1, which is
quite likely, then you are dealing with a double blow to your moisture
levels. A deficiency in histidine also leaves eczema patients vulnerable to
higher levels of histamine and greater allergic tendencies.

The stratum granulosum should function as a second skin barrier due
to the tight junctions forming between the cells. These junctions are
made of a complex of binding and building proteins, a bit like cemen-
ting bricks together within a scaffolding structure. The structure enables the skin to control and regulate the evaporation of water and
the passing of ions and solutes through cell pathways. (Ions are otherwise known as electrolytes; common examples are potassium, calcium, sodium etc., and solutes are just these electrolytes dissolved in
a watery solution in the skin). The tight junctions formed with the
claudin-1 protein should also continue to play an essential role in controlling the invasion of viruses, bacteria, and potential allergens. If these
junctions do not form effectively, as is the case with eczematous skin,
invaders can penetrate the skin more easily and trigger an immune or
allergy response in the dermis layer.

Some invading pathogenic organisms can directly break into your
cells. Others can alter the structure of the tight junctions by inserting
effectors, which are so-called because they can exert direct effects on
how the tight junctions operate, almost like hijacking them. They can
also activate different signals within your skin cells, changing their
behaviour or even directly connecting to them. The result of all these
is partial breaks in the junctions, allowing the skin to become more
permeable to pathogens. (39) Some pathogenic invaders, particularly
Staphylococcus, are so inflammatory they are given the term super-an-
tigens because they trigger a hyper-immune response. When you bear
in mind that people with eczema have lower levels of antibacterial protection on their skin through a lack of sebum and natural moisturizing
factor (which means they have higher levels of pathogens like *Staphylococcus*), these breaks in the skin barrier junctions mean eczema patients

are set up for an ambush of *Staphylococcus* invasions and the subsequent inflammation caused by the immune system hyper-reacting.

Going back to the skin layers, another event that occurs in this third layer is the destruction of the nucleus (the brain or factory of your cells) and all their organelles (minute cell organs) within the keratinocytes to make room for more keratin. This is very similar to what your red blood cells do; they also start with a nucleus but destroy it to make more room to carry oxygen. Without a nucleus, these cells can no longer reproduce or form any intracellular functions. Filling up with keratin to their maximum capacity enables the cells to later provide the tough outer coating necessary at the surface of the skin. This is especially important for skin protection. If the body cannot form enough keratin proteins for the cells to absorb, this will affect their ability to become effective hard corneocytes (dead skin cells) at the outer layer of your skin. This will also make the skin more susceptible to invasions by pathogens and allergens and become a third contributor to excessive water evaporation.

In healthy skin, those tight junctions between the cells formed in the previous basale layer enable the stratum granulosum to function as an effective second barrier. However, in eczematous skin, these processes are breaking down, and the skin is not forming correctly. Consequently, the barriers are not forming effectively either.

The keratinocytes in this layer are now too far from the dermis to be able to receive nutrients and oxygen from the blood supply, so as they move into the final layer, the stratum corneum, they undergo a specific process of cell death.

In the stratum corneum, the tight junction proteins should still control the selective permeability of the epidermis skin layer and, consequently, the barrier function. As the cells move into this layer, an action occurs in healthy skin, which is yet another major breakdown in eczematous skin. A protease enzyme acts on a substance called profilaggrin. (This is another protein carried in the cells toward the surface of the skin), to convert it into a different form of the protein called filaggrin. This vital action causes the cells to collapse like an umbrella, resulting in several important biproducts. Firstly, as the cells collapse, their remains become tough flat cells called corneocytes. These are the harder, dead, flat skin cells that form the outer layer of our skin, the final external barrier. Secondly, the remaining filaggrin in the cells, along with the amino acids (proteins) such as arginine, glutamine, and histidine, create the natural moisturizing element of the skin. The lipids (fats) contained in the cell spill out and surround the corneocytes (the collapsed dead cells) to keep them waterproof and supple, and the water that was held by the histidine is released into the spaces of the epidermal cells to keep the skin moist. This layer of water and fats is known as the natural moisturizing factor. It has a pivotal role in keeping the skin healthy, moist, supple, and protected from external irritants, partly by restricting the evaporation of water out from the skin and partly by blocking the ingress of irritants into the skin. Thirdly, these same amino acids generate the production of two essential biproducts called urocanic acid and 5-pyrrolidone carboxylic acid. These substances are natural antibacterial agents and have been shown to inhibit the growth of *Staphylococcus aureus* in the skin. (2,39) anyone with eczema would likely be familiar with *Staphylococcus* because it is one of the most common bacterial infections to afflict eczematous skin. In fact, studies have shown a direct correlation between the extent of *Staphylococcus* colonization on a patient's skin and the severity of their eczema. I will talk more about the effects of *Staphylococcus* in Chapter 7.

Despite having all these layers, which totals around 40-45 layers of cells, the entire epidermis is only 0.1 mm thick. That is around the same thickness as a sheet of paper, which is amazing. The complete process of skin renewal from the stratum basale to the stratum corneum takes around 45 days. It is a constant process, which is encouraging because it means any action we take now to improve the quality of our skin from within will produce evidenced results at the surface within about six weeks.

Are you now seeing how the eczema rash is caused by defects in the production of new skin? Let me show you, with two of my own sketches, the differences between healthy and eczematous skin. I have not drawn all the layers, just enough to represent what it should look like. Remember, it is around 45 layers thick. (I know these pictures are crude, but I use these in my courses, and they serve to illustrate my point quite effectively, especially regarding the protein deficiencies affecting the ability of your body to produce efficient skin layers.)

Healthy skin should look something like this:

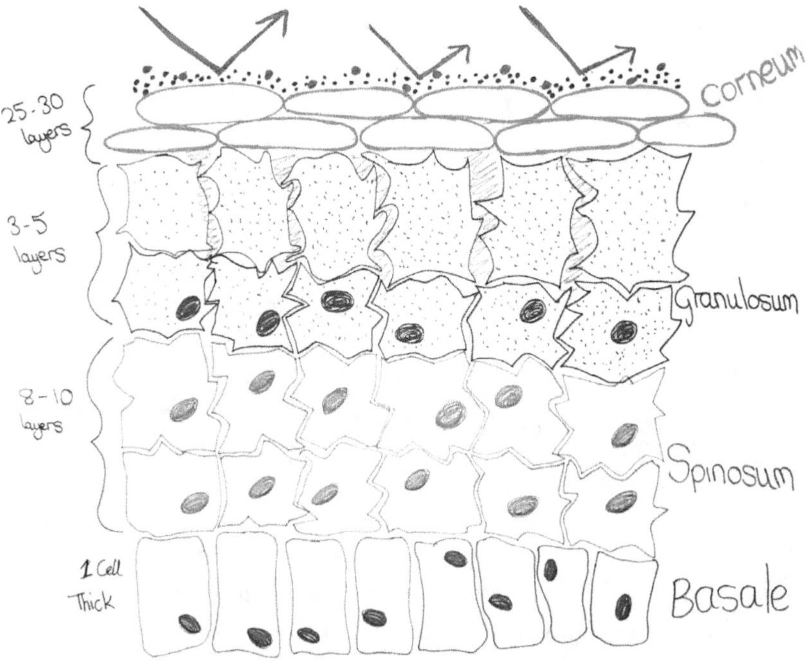

The smallest dots on the surface represent robust colonies of friendly microbes, and the larger red dots, the *Staphylococcus* bacterium, which is kept under control by the skin microbes. Irritants and allergens are prevented from entering the skin by the tight junctions and the natural moisturizing factors.

Now, in contrast, instead of the strong, healthy, tightly knitted skin layers shown in this picture above, eczematous skin looks more like this:

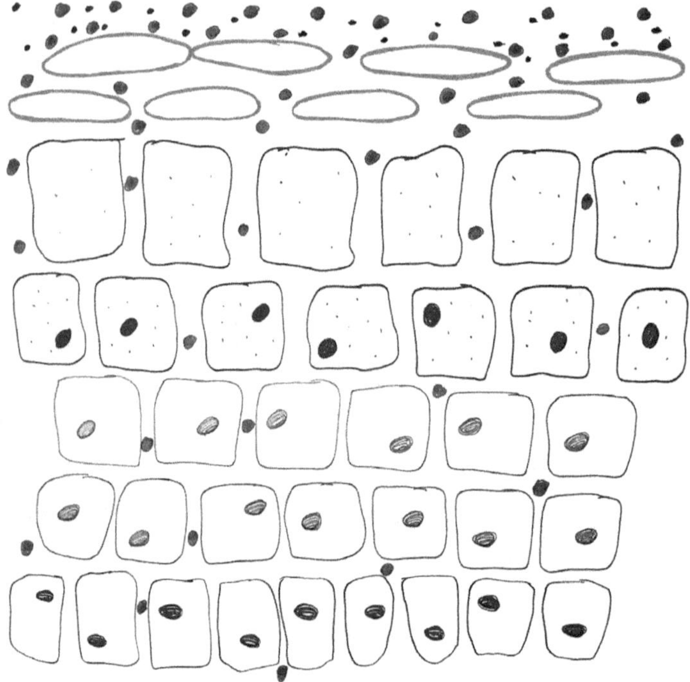

What is different? The tight junctions have not formed, there are fewer keratohyalin granules inside the cells, less histidine proteins to carry water in the cells, fewer lipids for waterproof protection, and insufficient enzyme and protein functions. Consequently, the collapsing of cells and formation of an effective corneum layer barrier function become disrupted. This allows irritants and allergens to ingress the skin more easily. There are also fewer friendly microbes residing on the skin (the tiny dots on the top layer) and less natural moisturizing factor. As a result, pathogenic bacteria (the larger dots on the surface) can flourish, overpopulate, and start invading below the skin's surface to penetrate the very bottom layer of the epidermis and enter the dermis, where your immune cells lie in wait for invaders.

Let us summarize what we have discovered so far. In our review, we have identified the following differences in the formation of eczematous skin compared to healthy skin.

1. A deficiency in claudin-1 protein, which detrimentally affects the ability to produce the tight junctions that protect the skin from the invasions of bacteria, fungus, and allergens, and allows water to evaporate at a much faster rate than normal, leaving the skin too dry. Instead of the skin being like interlocking bricks in the skin wall, eczematous skin is like a wall built with disconnected bricks and minimal cement. Consequently, the wall is very weak.

2. There is also a deficiency in histidine, which should bind to and carry water in the cells up through the skin layers, keeping the skin moist. This contributes to excessively dry skin. In addition, histidine regulates the action of histamine in allergic responses. It is also involved in efficiently converting profilaggrin to filaggrin and the umbrella-like collapse of the cells to form the hard, exterior barrier. With low levels of histidine, your skin cannot make an effective final barrier layer, nor can it regulate your histamine, leaving you vulnerable to higher-than-normal levels, making you more prone to allergic responses.

3. A lack of natural moisturizing factor means your skin has less natural moisturizing oil, less water content, and lower antibacterial protection, allowing the pathogenic bacteria on your skin to overpopulate. (2) As you have not created effective tight junctions, there are abnormal spaces between the skin cells, which enable pathogens (and other potential allergens) to penetrate between the cells and enter the dermal layer below, setting off an immune response.

4. An inefficient outer skin layer due to the combination of breakdowns, and the ineffective collapse of the keratinocytes into the hard corneocyte layer, allowing excess water evaporation and a tendency to produce new skin that is already dry and over-sensitive.

5. Possible deficiencies in other proteins such as keratin to make tough skin cells, collagen to produce effective adhesions between the cells and in the tight junctions, and arginine and glutamine, which are necessary for an effective natural moisturizing factor.

This is all eye-opening information, but it is still not the root cause of eczema. We need to peel back the onion layers further and look deeper to find out WHY these issues are occurring. However, in the meantime, you can take some simple steps to start supporting your body and to help it function more efficiently, which is what I will explain next.

Firstly though, as I have mentioned essential skin proteins such as claudin 1, histidine, filaggrin, and keratin, let me quickly explain why these proteins are so crucial.

When we think of protein, we often think of meat, such as a piece of steak. However, proteins are an integral part of plant-based foods too. All proteins, including those found in steaks, are made of amino acids, which are like Lego bricks; how you fit them together determines what you can build. You can take apart a Lego building, change how you fit the pieces together, and make something completely different with the same bricks. In the same way, when we consume protein, whether from an animal or plant source, our body digests it and breaks it down into its simplest form: amino acids. Your cells then follow the instructions in your DNA code to build whatever proteins it needs from your available amino acids. These proteins are used for a myriad of functions in the body, such as growth, repair, skin production, enzymes, and immune function, to name a few. Some amino acids can be made in the body, but others cannot. The ones your body cannot make are called essential amino acids, which must be obtained regularly from the diet. Histidine was never previously considered an essential amino acid; however, many experts are now including it in the list as multitudes of people now display a reduced capacity to produce it effectively in their bodies.

There are many reasons why you may be deficient in proteins, not only poor nutrition. We will examine these in subsequent chapters, but for now, the important thing to note is that you can provide your body with additional amino acids by direct supplementation.

A group of scientists published a study in 2017 reporting that they achieved a significant improvement in the skin of adult eczema patients by supplementing them with 4 grams of L-histidine once daily. After only four weeks, the skin had improved to a level comparable to the use of mid-potency corticosteroids but without any side effects. (1) The study concluded that L-histidine supplementation was a safe and effective treatment option for eczema patients. I highly recommend that you print a copy of this study and take it to your doctor to read. L-histidine can be purchased alone or in an amino acid complex. I recommend finding a source of organic aminos that includes all nine essential amino acids. I use a plant-based amino acid product made from organic pea protein to make a protein shake every day; however, some people are allergic to pea protein and will not be able to tolerate this. If you purchase beef or whey protein (subject to your food sensitivities), ensure it is organic and non-GMO, the reason for which I will expound on later. Amino acids can also be purchased as pharmaceutical-grade supplements or hypoallergenic formula milk. These options can be more suitable for children and adults with multiple allergies, and often find it challenging to find safe aminos (particularly in the case of eosinophilic disease). If you have an issue synthesizing or producing histidine, it is highly likely you will have a similar problem with other amino acids too. Hence why I recommend taking supplements of all essential amino acids, not just histidine. Just be sure to check that the histidine content is sufficiently high enough to make a difference and if necessary, take an additional amount of L-Histidine to get to the 4-gram dose recommended for adults) in the study. For children, it is commonly accepted that the dosage should be proportionate to the child's weight. Therefore, if a standard adult weight is 160 lbs., and the adult dose is 4000 mg (4 g), then a 40-lb child should take one-quarter of the adult dose, which equates to 1000 mg (1 g). However, this should be done in conjunction with your doctor. I reiterate I am not a qualified medical professional. I am sharing information with you that I have found in the published scientific literature for you to take to your doctor. If your doctor is unwilling to act on evidence-based science documents, you may need to look for a different doctor who will. (A growing number of qualified medical professionals have undergone additional training in how food, nutrition, and lifestyle impact our health. As a generalization, these doctors are more open to receiving scientific studies they may not have seen before. They are often called functional or integrative medicine professionals.)

With regards to the lack of natural moisturizing factor, this is a deep rabbit hole by itself, with lots of information to note; therefore, I have devoted the next chapter solely to this issue. Together with this chapter, they make up the teaching on the first spider leg. I will also show you effective ways to restore the natural antibacterial protection of your skin to overcome the lack of natural moisturizing factor. We can then move on to Chapter 6, where we can examine the next spider leg; the reasons why your body is not producing skin proteins as effectively as people without eczema.

Actions Points

1. Take pure L-histidine supplemental powder at a dose of 4 g, taken once daily in the morning, mixed in juice.
2. Consider adding an organic protein powder to supplement other essential amino acids (ensure that you check the ingredients for known allergens).

5

Ditching the Itch

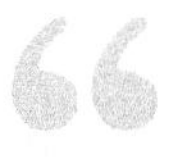 *There are simple, effective, external measures one can take to help alleviate the dryness quickly. Some of them are so straightforward and easy to implement, I never cease to be amazed why patients are not given these tips by their doctors or consultants!"*

Lack of sebum is usually the most common cause given on the 'diagnosis' of eczema. As we have already identified, a lack of sebum means the skin lacks moisture and has an impaired barrier function. This is the simple explanation, and although it does not consider the myriad of other factors causing eczema or identify that natural moisturising factor and sebum are not the same thing, the resulting dry skin is still a big issue. Therefore, we must look at ways to reduce the dryness and consequent itching. Scratching causes damage to the already weakened barrier and allows even more bacteria and allergens to gain access below the skin surface. There are simple, effective, external measures one can take to help quickly alleviate the dryness. Some of them are so straightforward and easy to implement I never cease to be amazed that patients are not given these tips by their doctors or consultants. It would save patients a great deal of suffering.

Firstly, let me recap what sebum is, and then we will take a deeper look at why the antibacterial protection deficiencies cause such a problem.

Sebum is considered a component of the natural moisturising factor of the skin. It provides the waxy/oily substance that creates an occlusive or waterproof film on top of the skin and helps to limit water evaporation from the epidermis layer. It stands to reason that having a deficient sebum level would allow more water than normal to evaporate from the skin, leaving it overly dry. However, it has a knock-on effect of defective processing within the skin layers.

When something goes awry with the processing of profilaggrin to filaggrin and the collapse of cells, the natural moisturising factor is reduced, and the hard flat corneocytes are not formed correctly, leaving the final exterior layer too weak to perform its protective function effectively. Excessive dryness then leaves the skin itchy, resulting in mechanical injury as a direct consequence of scratching. Having a weakened, dry skin barrier means that the skin is more detrimentally affected by physical irritation, such as hot water, sweat, and ultraviolet exposure, for example. All of these can further weaken the epidermal barrier and trigger eczema flares. They can also result in the development of non-specific hypersensitivities of the skin towards many other kinds of irritant factors, such as woollen clothing, tobacco smoke, and physical factors like cold, heat, and even washing. (16)

As mentioned earlier, sebum also contains antibacterial agents, such as urocanic acid and 5-pyrrolidone carboxylic acid. These help to regulate the colonies of microbes in the skin. Reduced sebum levels leave the skin with lower antibacterial protection levels and, consequently, a higher risk of colonisation by harmful, pathogenic microbes. These pathogenic infections are a common feature of eczema rashes, triggering inflammation and irritation. (6) Reduced antibacterial protection allows for the over-colonisation of pathogens such as *Staphylococcus aureus, Staphylococcus epidermidis, Escherichia coli, Acinetobacter baumanii,* and *Pseudomonas aeruginosa* in addition to Candida albicans and Malassezia Furfur (types of yeast pathogen). These pathogens are all known to cause eczema when allowed to proliferate. (112) Without having effective tight junctions, these pathogens can penetrate the skin, which results in an increased inflammatory response, meaning more flare-ups and more itching. As previously mentioned, there is a direct correlation between the number of *Staphylococcus* in the skin and the severity of a person's eczema. This is likely due to the *Staphylococcus* releasing particularly nasty toxins into the skin called enterotoxins. Your immune cells pick up these enterotoxins and recognise them as being from a dangerous invader. Enterotoxins are so inflammatory that they trigger what is called a superantigen effect (meaning they result in an overly excessive activation of the immune system, causing the release of massive amounts of cytokines, which further drive the inflammatory cycle). More than 50% of *Staphylococcus aureus* isolates cultured in a lab from patients with eczema were seen to have the ability to produce these enterotoxins and the resulting superantigen effect. *Staphylococcus* enterotoxin B is so inflammatory that it has even been shown to cause a dermatitis rash after being applied to normal healthy skin. (16) Thus, it does not take a rocket scientist to realise how much inflammation it will cause to eczematous skin that allows for faster and deeper penetration through the skin layers.

Eczema patients are not only prone to developing more *Staphylococcus* infections but also to a variety of other skin diseases of fungal, viral, or bacterial origin, such as candida, eczema herpeticum, and *Staphylococcal impetigo*. Scientists have investigated whether defective immunity is a potential reason for this, in addition to the reduced antibacterial action of the sebum. (16) However, the problem is more likely due to the inability to create an effective skin barrier and natural moisturising factor. The immune system is defective in eczema, but, as you will see in a later chapter, this is a consequence of the skin barrier defects causing inflammatory cycles that need to be interrupted to break free from eczema. It is one of the loops in the spider web I mentioned at the beginning of the book. In Chapter 7, we examine the immune responses involved in the mechanisms of eczema and how to break the cycles.

Hopefully, you can now see why sebum and natural moisturising factor are so crucial to the health of our skin and why it is imperative that we try to combat their deficiency. So the question is: What can we do to help alleviate the excessive dryness of your skin and the loss of antibacterial protection? There are many actions you can take.

Back in 2008, studies began investigating whether hard water was an exacerbating factor in eczema. (106, 107) Water hardness was found to be positively correlated with eczema development and severity. I repeat that was back in 2008. As I write this book, well over a decade later, I am dismayed how few eczema patients are still not being advised to check the water hardness in their area or to fit a water softener. It really does exacerbate eczema, and it is one of the first things you need to check if you seek to protect the moisture levels in your skin.

What is hard water? Hard or soft water is determined by the minerals in the ground that the water flows through. The higher the concentrations of these minerals, particularly calcium and magnesium in the form of sulphates, the harder the water becomes and the more drying it is to the skin. People with healthy skin may not notice any detrimental effects of bathing in hard water, but eczema patients already experiencing reduced natural moisture levels will find their condition significantly worsened by it.

After finding out about hard water, I checked with my local water supplier, and sure enough, we lived in an area with hard water. Following some research, I purchased a limescale control device for my household, hopeful that its claims to use an electrical charge to change the minerals and soften the water would help my children. However, very disappointingly, we saw zero beneficial effects on their skin. From the point of view of eczema management, it was a total failure, and I returned the product to the company. Sometime later, I saw an advertisement for a salt block water softener, which promised to alleviate dry skin. Despite being let down by the previous electric version, I decided to try it. The effect on my children's skin was incredible! Although it did not completely heal them, if you asked me to name the measure with the fastest results on my children's skin, I would tell you it was installing the water softener. I was left wondering why I had not been told about such a simple action by my doctor. It is now one of the first things I tell eczema patients to do. Very few patients are aware of the exacerbating effects of hard water, and yet it can be mitigated by spending only a small amount of money each month. I say 'small' because the benefits to your skin are easily worth the price; however, in addition to the skin health pros, the cost is recouped easily through the increased foaming effects of soft water compared to hard. This means you need to use less soap products, shampoo, and laundry detergents to achieve the same cleaning results, reducing your bills for buying these products. Softened water also does not leave limescale in your pipes and around sinks. Thus, a water softener helps to prolong the life of your kettle, iron, washing machine, and dishwasher. For those people with central heating, your boiler, pipes, and radiators, too, as there will be less build-up of limescale deposits inside them, meaning energy bills will also be dramatically reduced. If you are wondering where to purchase a softener, I recommend contacting Monarch Water in the United Kingdom. I recently partnered with them to increase awareness of the benefits of water softeners for eczema sufferers. Their prices are very competitive. They are high quality, and their softeners are Water Regulations Advisory Scheme approved. I was impressed by Monarch because they stand by their products, giving a 7-year labour warranty in addition to their 2-year part warranty in the United Kingdom. I do not know any other water softener companies that offer that. Although they do not sell direct to the public, if you email them (info@monarchwater.co.uk) and quote "The Eczema Channel" (my YouTube Channel), they will happily connect you with your local supplier and, in addition, enter you into a draw to potentially win £50 worth of 'Love2Shop' vouchers (current value at the time of writing this book).

A further water treatment I recommend is either a whole-house water filtration system if your budget permits or a chlorine filter to fit onto the shower head, at the very least, if your budget cannot stretch to the whole-house version.

Chlorine was first added to public drinking water systems in the 19th century as a disinfectant. Consequently, many water-borne diseases were significantly reduced. It then became common practice to add chlorine to all public water systems in general, starting in Maidstone, England, in 1897. However, while it helped to reduce the incidence of water-related diseases, it is not beneficial to bathe in. Chlorine attacks any organic matter, meaning anything that lives; this not only includes pathogenic bacteria, but also your skin, the mucus membranes of your eyes, nose, mouth, and lungs, and of course, the precious microbiome that resides both on and in us. (Have you ever had stinging red eyes after swimming in a chlorinated swimming pool? This is the reason why.)

The Food Revolution Network published an article on chlorine in drinking water and cited a report from the United States Council of Environmental Quality. It stated: "The cancer risk for people who drink chlorinated water is up to 93% higher than for those whose water does not contain chlorine." It further stated, from the same source, that "Americans now consume between 300-600 times the amount of chlorine that is considered safe." Yikes!

In addition, chlorine also has a drying effect on the skin and has been positively linked to both a greater risk of developing eczema and to increased severity. (106, 107) However, it is relatively easy to remove. We purchased a low-cost shower water filter that was fitted before the shower head and effectively removed over 99% of the chlorine from our shower water. When I filled the bath for the children, I filled it from the shower rather than the taps to ensure that their water was also clear from chlorine contamination. We replaced the chlorine filter every six months. (I will address the consequences of decimating our microbiomes with chlorine and other means in Chapter 9.)

The reason I recommend a whole-house filter over a chlorine filter alone is that many municipal water supplies have other toxins in the water. For example, houses built many years ago can have deteriorating lead pipes that leach lead contamination into the water supply. Furthermore, other pollutants such as pesticides and estrogen can find their way into water reservoirs and, consequently, our taps. Many of these contaminants (which I discuss in Chapter 12) are directly implicated in eczema development. Thus, a better solution is to install a whole house system, if possible, to remove them. Monarch can also help you with water filtration systems. Please email them at: info@monarch.co.uk, remembering to quote The Eczema Channel.

Other measures can help to address the effects of dryness and external irritants, which are also quite easy to implement. Firstly, moisturising the skin frequently with skin-nourishing moisturisers is imperative. I say 'skin nourishing' because not all moisturisers are equal. Some contain nutrients that aid the skin's regeneration, and some hinder it. Check the products you are using. If they contain sodium lauryl sulphate, I recommend you ditch them as quickly as possible. Sodium lauryl sulphate is a common ingredient in prescribed emollients such as aqueous creams and other personal care products. They bind to the proteins in the skin, hindering the formation of an effective corneum layer. People with eczema show a significantly lower threshold of irritation from sodium lauryl sulphate than those with healthy skin. (91) It also strips the skin of natural moisture, further exacerbating the problem of dry skin. Studies show that sodium lauryl sulphate disrupts the barrier function of the cornified cell layer. (14) In addition, sodium lauryl sulphate has been shown to cause allergic reactions resulting in rashes, which is why prescribing it to use on eczematous skin is ridiculously counterproductive. It is crucial to avoid chemical-based soaps when trying to heal from eczema as they can disrupt the acid mantle of the skin, which will contribute to even more excessive drying and compromise the natural antibacterial and antifungal protection of the skin. Acid and alkaline strengths are measured on a pH scale with 1 being the strongest acid and 7 being neutral. The higher the number, the more alkaline the substance. Healthy skin is naturally at a pH of 5.5 to 6, which is slightly acidic. Alkaline soaps will affect the skin's pH, stripping down its natural acid mantle, which helps protect it from bacteria and fungus, consequently leaving it more prone to infection than it already is. Natural oil-based soaps, such as those made from coconut or shea, do not dry the skin in the same way and are much preferable.

It is important to realise that not all people respond to products in the same way, so my rule of thumb is to check your skin after you bathe. If your skin feels drier and tauter than usual after using a product, do not use it. Instead, try to find something else that is less drying. We have found that using natural coconut-based soaps or natural non-drying body washes, such as Dr Bronner's liquid soap for sensitive skin or Lavera sensitive, combined with the water filter and water-softener, is far less drying. There are companies now making gentle organic products explicitly developed for eczematous skin, but please always remember to check the ingredient labels. Just because something says it is suitable for eczema or is natural does not mean it is ideal for you. Some may contain allergens like milk or nut products, and some that claim to be natural contain more chemicals than you can even pronounce.

One particularly soothing natural bath treatment for dry skin is to place organic porridge oats in a stocking and soak them in the bath water before bathing. When you squeeze the oats, they release a creamy moisturising substance into the bathwater, which resembles milk. It is very softening for dry skin, but I urge caution when using food substances in this way if the skin is open and raw. This is because there is a possibility of those food proteins passing through the damaged skin and causing an immune reaction which could trigger an allergic response when the food is eaten at a subsequent time. I will explain this in more detail in Chapter 8.

To moisturise, I used pure, unrefined shea butter on all my children. It worked beautifully and caused no reactions despite their medical consultant informing me that I should not use it because three of my children had nut allergies. Look for pure, unrefined virgin shea butter, as it still contains skin-friendly nutrients in contrast to processed and refined versions, where the nutrients have been destroyed. Shea butter is very thick. If you live in a warm climate, it softens enough to spread quite readily, but in colder climates, such as winter in the United Kingdom, it will become too thick to apply without pulling on the skin. Please remember it can be painful to spread thick creams across damaged skin. I gently melted my shea butter in a glass bowl sitting over a pot of hot water. Once softened, I added jojoba oil (approximately 1:4 ratio of jojoba to shea butter) and mixed them together. Then I would cool the mixture, stirring it a few times as it cooled to ensure it did not separate. This creates a softer version, which is easier to spread. You can also buy ready-whipped versions that still retain their virgin unrefined properties but have been made softer to enable easier moisturising. Shea butter has only been studied in small-scale trials; nonetheless, the results show it to be much more effective as an emollient than commercial or pharmaceutical eczema products. After only 1 week of use, it led to greater levels of improvement in both skin smoothness and comfort. (105) You can purchase natural unrefined shea butter at a lower cost from companies that purchase directly from local producers in countries such as Ghana and then sells them direct to the public. I purchased online from a company called Akoma Skincare in Derby, in the United Kingdom. If you like natural ingredients and are interested in purchasing the raw materials to make your own products, you will love browsing their website. An alternative version for anyone who finds they cannot use shea butter is mango butter. It is made from the smaller seed inside the hard mango stone and has also been reported to be helpful for eczema and psoriasis. You can use mango butter in the same way as shea butter.

For one of my children, I did need to use a pharmaceutical emollient called Dermol Cream for a while. At that time, she suffered from severe eczema and had repeated skin infections of *Staphylococcus*, causing large puss-filled boils. Back then, I had yet to learn all the information I am currently passing on to you, so I went with the available options. Dermol cream is antimicrobial, so we used this for a short period to effectively manage the *Staphylococcus* and bring it under control. It can be used as both a soap substitute and a moisturiser. Not everyone can use Dermol Cream though; I know of many eczema patients who have suffered reactions to this product, so it is not something I recommend. In addition, Dermol Cream also indiscriminately kills friendly microbes, which creates further problems with skin microbial dysbiosis (friendly and pathogenic bacterium levels being out of balance) if used for too long. So along with the interventions we used to treat the other 'legs' of the eczema spider, I transitioned her to shea butter as her skin improved.

I have recently seen research about another product called ASEA, which uses a colourless, clear liquid derived from saline. Patented as MDI-P, it was seen to kill *Staphylococcus aureus, Pseudomonas aeruginosa, Legionella pneumophila,* and *Candida albicans* in laboratory tests, with no evidence of harm or tissue injury. If I had heard about ASEA when I struggled with skin infections in my children, I would have tried this product. You may want to consider looking into it. (113)

Whilst writing this book, we have been through a couple of years of Covid-19 restrictions and are still enduring some Covid-19 protocols.

One of these is the enforced sanitising of hands every time we enter a building. While there may be merits to killing pathogenic bacteria on our hands to avoid spreading germs, consistently using products that also decimate our healthy bacterial levels has led to an enormous increase in people developing hand eczema. The alcohol in sanitisers is also particularly drying, and excessive use causes the skin to crack open and allows bacteria, germs, and chemical irritants to enter. It is much better to find less drying and damaging products, and it would be worth checking ewg.org or your local health store for more skin-friendly and non-toxic options. A colloidal silver spray is an excellent option. You can also create your own antibacterial and antiviral moisturiser by adding a few drops of thyme essential oil to your favourite hand cream. Most shop owners would be quite understanding if you used your own sanitiser and can show that it is also antimicrobial but more suitable for eczema. You could also ask for a letter from your doctor if you prefer to carry proof of why you would rather not use alcohol-based sanitisers.

During this exceptionally challenging period dealing with my young daughter's eczema, her consultant prescribed cetirizine antihistamine. The intervention reduced her itching and allowed her skin some respite to recover from the mechanical injuries it had been repeatedly subjected to by constant scratching. Unfortunately, most of her body was covered by eczema at that point, and she was continually tormented by itching, especially at night. As a result, we were all sleep deprived and exhausted.

Cetirizine is not licensed for children under two years of age, and my daughter was only four months old when her consultant prescribed it. Although her consultant instructed me to keep her on cetirizine for two years, as soon as her skin had improved, which took around two months, I began to wean her off, gradually reducing her dose by imperceptible amounts every couple of days until she was no longer taking any antihistamine. By lowering her dose in stages, I did not cause any kickback reaction from having a sudden increase in her histamine levels due to reducing the antihistamines too rapidly. She never needed to return to daily antihistamine medications after that.

However, during the period she did use it, it was immensely helpful in giving her skin some respite and helping her to heal (as well as helping us to get some sleep when she was able to rest more comfortably).

To help the body mitigate the risk of pathogenic microbes over-colonising the skin, we need to take measures to address the reduced antibacterial protection of the skin due to insufficient sebum. There are several options to achieve this.

One of the most effective ways of restoring the skin's natural antibacterial balance is to spray probiotics directly onto the skin (along with supplementing with amino acids, as mentioned in the previous chapter). Doing this will help ensure that you begin producing an effective skin barrier and a more efficient natural moisturising factor.

Furthermore, adding Dead Sea salt to the bathwater is a much more effective protocol than antibacterial lotions. It has been scientifically proven that the rich magnesium salts present significantly improved skin barrier function, enhanced skin hydration levels, and reduced redness and inflammation. (88) The magnesium in Dead Sea salt differs from that in hard water. The former hydrates the skin; the latter dehydrates it. Magnesium sulphate in hard water is highly detrimental to eczema, whereas magnesium chloride in Dead Sea salt is beneficial. Thus, it is important to make the distinction that not all magnesium compounds are the same.

Another good thing to note is that salt does not kill the friendly *Lactobacillus* bacterial strain that naturally resides on the skin (which is why they also survive and flourish in homemade fermented veggies like Sauerkraut). Another commonly used ingredient many people have found helpful is adding a little raw apple cider vinegar to the bath water twice a week.

While we are on the topic of microbes, please allow me to vent some frustration while I explain something important. As a sweeping generalisation, humans have a natural propensity to be destructive rather than constructive. Consequently, we tend to overreact to any so-called invaders. Whether at war with nations, terrorists, diseases, or microbes, our reaction has historically been to blast the lot of them without considering the lasting damage caused to the environment and innocent bystanders. Take nuclear or chemical weapons as an example; they effectively annihilate enemies but also decimate civilians and, as a byproduct, create a toxic environment for many years to come. In the case of cancer treatment, the protocol is to annihilate the cancerous cells with chemical toxins or radiation, regardless of the destruction caused to the rest of the healthy cells in the tissues, immune system, and microbiome. Antibiotics are prescribed like candy to kill infections, but at the same time, they wipe out entire species of gut microbes and consequently damage the ability of the body to function optimally. Similarly, with the treatment of viruses and bacteria that we fear may infect us, we blast our skin with antibacterial washes, emollients, and sanitisers to help us feel safe; however, in the process, we decimate the natural antibacterial protection of our own commensurate microbes. Pathogens such as *Staphylococcus* and yeast tend to be more robust and recover their populations far more rapidly. Therefore, whether it be on the skin, in the gut, or elsewhere in the body, by following the 'blast them all' philosophy, we end up caught in a cycle of wiping out microbes indiscriminately, then having to use more antibiotics and sanitisers to treat the proliferation of pathogens that take over as a result. For this reason, I DO NOT advocate taking chlorine or bleach baths to treat eczema flares. I have already spoken about chlorine and its effects on the skin. If you take bleach baths, you are following the 'blast them all' system and will find yourself needing bleach baths more and more frequently as the *Staphylococcus* takes an even greater stronghold over your skin microbiome. A far more effective method of overcoming pathogens is to nurture and support the body's natural protectors by flooding the body with commensurate microbes, which can then crowd out and overcome pathogens, thus repairing and strengthening the natural innate immunity. This method is more about treating the underlying deficiencies that caused the overpopulation of pathogens in the first place and restoring equilibrium rather than fighting indiscriminately without thought to the consequences. We can do this by supporting the skin's natural microbiome and antibacterial properties. An effective way to do this is to use a probiotic powder mixed with water to spray onto the skin. One that has been shown to help in studies is *Lactobacillus rhamno-susmucosa*, which would naturally be present on healthy skin but is lacking in eczematous skin. Numerous topical probiotics are available to purchase now; some have been specifically designed for skin issues such as eczema and psoriasis. I also know of many people who have tried oral probiotics over the years for purposes other than their advertised intent and have seen them work wonders. Protocols range from diluting and spraying them over the skin before moisturising to gargling them to treat sore throats to even putting them on a clean tampon and inserting it to beat recurring vaginal thrush. There are many great probiotics on the market, which can be found online or at your local health store. As a generalisation, independent health stores tend to stock a broader range of high-quality supplements, including probiotics. I hope you understand my reasoning when I tell eczema patients to spray natural probiotics on the skin to restore the natural microbiome instead of blasting all known microbes off the terrain of their skin. Does it make sense? If it does, then I have successfully made my point.

Essential oils can also help manage bacterium levels. In a Greek study, the most effective essential oil against *Staphylococcus* was found to be thyme oil; it was so effective that it killed the *Staphylococcus* entirely in only 60 minutes. (104) Another study found that thyme oil was effective against ALL pathogens known to cause eczema, followed closely by lavender oil. Thyme oil mixes well with lavender and also with geranium. Others are still effective, although they are not quite so rapid in their efficacy. Tea tree is also antibacterial and effective against *Staphylococcus*, but do not use this around your pets, especially dogs, as it can be toxic for them to inhale.

One of my favourite concoctions is to mix equal amounts of eucalyptus oil, peppermint oil, and geranium oil into a small bottle of olive or coconut oil; five drops of each into 50 ml of carrier oil makes a very pleasant-smelling antibacterial, antiviral moisturiser to carry in your bag and repeatedly apply to dry patches throughout the day. (I also drip the same oils, in the same proportions, into a steam diffuser to clear the air if someone visits who appears to display any symptoms of a viral infection such as the common cold or influenza. As a result, no one in my household has caught any viruses bought in.) If you are not used to using essential oils, I recommend you try a patch test first with some *diluted* oil to ensure that they do not cause any reactions in your skin.

The final simple measure to reduce bacterial overload is to wash bedding, towels, and as many items as possible on a hot wash and tumble dry on high heat (providing you will not shrink them - please check your laundry labels). Despite people advocating that sunlight kills dust mites, I do not recommend drying laundry outside when you have eczematous skin. This is because outdoor allergens such as pollen can attach to the laundry and enter the skin through the eczema lesions encouraging a hypersensitive reaction, which can cause allergic responses on subsequent exposure to the pollen. An alternative method to kill dust mites is to freeze items for a few hours in the day or overnight. So, if you have items or soft toys that you cannot launder on a hot cycle, this is another option. One thing to mention that is imperative with laundry: do not use biological washing powders as the enzymes can cause allergic reactions that cause eczema to flare up. Only use non-biological laundry soap and avoid fabric softeners, tumble-drying fresheners, and scents. Fabric softeners typically contain quaternary ammonium compounds, which are used to reduce static electricity but are known to cause skin and respiratory irritation. It is one of the five most common chemical skin irritants. Other chemical additives known to cause skin reactions are methylisothiazolinone, its derivatives, and formaldehyde-releasing compounds. I discuss these further in Chapter 12 when we examine the involvement of toxins in eczema.

Many chemicals in detergents and biological laundry soaps are known to exacerbate eczema. (64, 102, 108) Therefore, it is advisable to avoid chemical products. Eco-friendly products are much safer for everyone in the family as the chemical exposure from detergents is quite high. However, if you use standard laundry soaps, perhaps those designed for sensitive skin, use an extra rinse option on the washing machine to ensure that you rinse out as much of the potentially reactive chemicals as possible.

We looked earlier at how certain proteins are required to produce healthy skin. The body makes these proteins from amino acids. Several things can affect the efficient manufacture of these proteins, and we will look at these in detail later in the book. However, the important thing for you to know about these proteins now is that you can assist your body by providing it with additional amino acids in a form that the body can assimilate quickly. This will also help you to produce a more effective natural moisturising factor. L-histidine supplements have been shown to be incorporated into profilaggrin and released into the natural moisturising factor as soon as 1 day after consumption. Even the slowest result, which was reported to be seven days, is still remarkably swift for something with no detrimental side effects. (1, 14)

We are now starting to draw our eczema spider web. The first strand of the web is in place; dermatology, or lack of natural moisturising factor. As we go through the chapters, we will add the other legs, enabling you to see how the legs interact and drive the disease state.

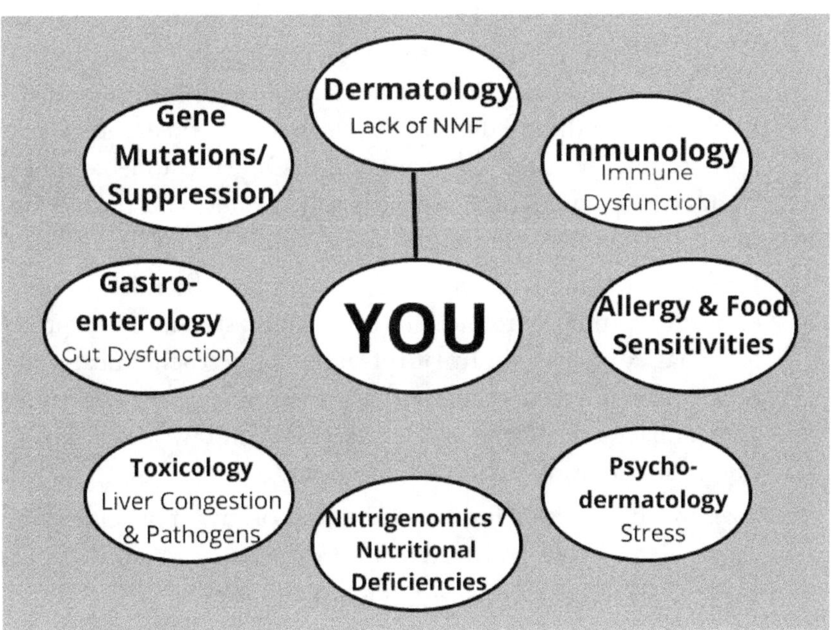

To summarise, these are the action points from this chapter that you should implement as soon as possible to restore and support a healthier natural moisturising factor. Now that we have completed our discussion of this topic let us go deeper and look at WHY eczema patients cannot manufacture the skin proteins they require effectively.

Action points

1. If necessary, check your water supply and fit a water softener, ensuring you use the block salt version.

2. Fit a water filtration system that includes a drinking water solution, preferably a whole-house filter. If funds do not permit, purchase a chlorine shower filter and countertop drinking water filter instead. If using a shower chlorine filter, fill baths from the shower rather than the taps to ensure that the bath water is also free from chlorine.

3. Launder clothes using HOT water and dry them on a HIGH HEAT. (Please remember to check the laundry labels on the items you are washing. You do not want to shrink your clothes.) Avoid outdoor drying during the pollen season. Freeze items that cannot be hot-washed to kill dust mites. Only use non-biological laundry soaps, preferably eco-friendly brands, and do not use fabric softeners or laundry fresheners.

4. Find a natural moisturising product with skin-friendly ingredients, such as pure unrefined shea butter and stop using all products that contain sodium lauryl sulphate, petrochemicals, and other unhelpful ingredients. Adding essential oils can effectively control bacterium levels, but be careful with raw, open skin in case of sensitisation or allergic reactions.

5. Soak in a bath with a little Dead Sea salt or raw apple cider vinegar added to your bathwater twice a week.

6. Spray probiotics onto your skin before moisturising.

The Weakest Link

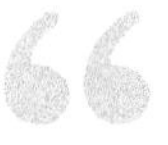

Right from the beginning of life when a baby forms in the womb, cell division occurs, and portions of the DNA code are activated to determine what happens next."

Who remembers the game show The Weakness Link, which first aired in April 2001? It was hosted by Anne Robinson and had contestants competing and voting out the weakest link in the chain until only one was left standing. Although our genes do not compete and vote each other out like in the game show, every one of us has weak links in the form of genetic mutations. WHERE your weakest links are can play a significant role in determining your susceptibility to developing certain diseases.

When comparing healthy skin to eczematous skin, there are marked changes that can be caused by genetic mutations. In 1990, a team of international scientists jointly embarked on the most extensive international gene project to map the entire human genome and identify what each gene codes for. It took 13 years to complete (2003), which was two years ahead of schedule. The phenomenal work has enabled researchers to identify the genetic links to many diseases. This initially led to the belief that having specific 'disease genes' would result in us developing those diseases as an absolute certainty. Hence why, for example, multiple women who were identified as carrying the mutated BRCA1/2 genes opted to have preventative mastectomies to protect them from developing breast cancer. As the study of genetics has increased, it is becoming apparent that although a gene mutation may predispose a person to developing a disease, it is not an absolute given that the disease will occur. For example, scientists have studied identical twins whose genetic makeup is almost identical; they observed that while one twin may develop a disease for which they are genetically predisposed, the other twin does not. Therefore, it was found that other factors come into play, which are collectively studied in the relatively new field of science called epigenetics. Epigenetics looks at how gene expression or 'switches' are influenced by our environment and lifestyle, which is a fascinating development. Before we get into this, let us discuss genes and DNA.

Our cells start life with a nucleus, otherwise known as the brain of a cell. Our DNA code is the entire instruction manual of how to make us and how to perform all the maintenance issues and functions of our bodies. The DNA is stored in the nucleus of the cells. Mature red blood cells do not carry any DNA as these cells destroy their nucleus to enable more space for carrying oxygen around our body, much the same way our skin, nail, and hair cells make more room to fill up with keratin. Aside from these, all the other cells in our body contain a copy of our DNA.

As many cell types in our body are simultaneously undergoing a cycle of dying and being replaced, our DNA is constantly being copied. Every time a cell in our body replicates, it needs a complete copy of our DNA code or gene sequence. The code contains the entire 'instruction manual' of how to make us; this contains short coding sequences for making the proteins needed for repair and conducting all the processes in the body. The code sequences are like sections of an instruction manual directing cells on how to make proteins from amino acids.

Let us go back to our Lego illustration. Imagine you have a Lego building made from individual Lego bricks. If you dismantle the structure, you can use those bricks to build something with a completely different look and function, especially if you substitute different bricks from another batch of Lego. This is much like proteins. The protein sources in your diet are like the Lego buildings. First, your digestion breaks them down into amino acids (the individual bricks). Then your body uses the DNA code (the instruction manual) to build whatever protein (new Lego building) it needs from the available amino acids (bricks) in your body. Finally, the new structure is used to conduct the necessary processes for effective growth, function, and maintenance. These building and dismantling processes constantly occur within the cells in your body. At the end of each instruction or code sequence, there is a STOP codon, which informs the enzyme reading the DNA that the instruction has ended.

Your DNA code is so vital to your existence that it is kept safely wrapped up in a protective casing to shield it from damage. However, for the DNA to be copied, it must first be unzipped from its protective shell-like structure and unwound so that your enzymes can read it. In its unzipped state, DNA is extremely fragile and susceptible to damage from things like ultraviolet exposure, radiation, viruses, and certain chemicals and pollutants. As you can imagine, our DNA needs to be replicated constantly, so portions of unzipped, vulnerable DNA always exist.

Once the DNA is unwound, a polymerase enzyme (think of a specialist codebreaker) passes along the unravelled DNA and quickly copies the code in a process called transcription. (Transcribe means to copy a language into a written form so that it can be read.) This copy is called RNA. Occasionally, mistakes are made during the copying process, or if the DNA itself has been damaged, the enzyme will copy the error that resulted from the damage. Errors are referred to by different names depending on how they occurred. For example, some of the most common ones are:

DELETIONS occur when one or more bases (the individual characters of the code) have been accidentally omitted from the gene sequence.

INSERTIONS occur when the replication process accidentally inserts one or more additional bases that should not be there.

INVERSIONS mean one or more bases have effectively been switched around and are now in the wrong order.

SUBSTITUTIONS occur when one base is missing and has been substituted by an alternative base. If the substitution means the code now instructs for a totally different amino acid, it is called a missense mutation.

DUPLICATIONS are when a sequence of bases is duplicated too many times in error.

NONSENSE mutations are where the STOP codon (the "END of code" signal) has been inserted in the wrong place, effectively cutting short the instruction and preventing ANY amino acid from being made.

FRAMESHIFT mutations are where the start and/or stop codons are in the wrong place, causing an alteration in how the sequence of bases is read.

As you can see, many mistakes can be made in the process. Ultimately, these mutations result in abnormal protein formation, which often cannot effectively achieve the purpose for which it was initially required. (32)

When cells copy their DNA for cell replication, they must copy the complete instruction manual for each new cell. After the DNA is replicated to RNA, a second enzyme 'checks' the new strand for these errors and most often, they are found and corrected. However, if they are not, the changes will become part of the new DNA copy and will then become genetically inherited. Suppose any of the mutations permanently affect the ability of the cells to produce the correct proteins. In that case, they are called 'loss-of-function' mutations, and that portion of DNA can no longer code effectively for that specific function. (32) Uncorrected changes to any base sequences will change the instructions in that code and consequently change the outcome of whatever protein was being coded for. This will have the knock-on effect of the process the body needs that protein for not be performed efficiently. The three loss-of-function mutations particularly prevalent in eczema patients are missense, nonsense, and frameshifts.

As the body works together in one unit and is inextricably entwined, a mutation in one gene sequence can also affect or alter the expression of other genes. It is pretty scary when you think how vital these gene expressions are for our health.

In 2006, a breakthrough in understanding the genetics of eczema identified loss of function mutations within the epidermal differentiation complex. This is the area of our DNA that encodes skin proteins and is situated on chromosome 1. Simply put, there are 23 chromosome pairs in the human DNA. We inherited these chromosomes from our parents; one set from our biological mother and one from our biological father, which then pair. Each chromosome contains the instructions for coding the processes in specific body parts.

Studies in molecular genetics have shown that many gene mutations can be involved in eczema development. (16) Researchers from Mount Sinai School of Medicine, New York, used a tape-stripping method to remove skin cells for examination. They sought to identify the differences in the genes expressed (or switched on) in lesional eczema skin compared to normal skin. Shockingly, in eczema skin, they identified 2625 differentially expressed genes compared to normal skin. (35) Carrying mutations in this epidermal differentiation complex portion of chromosome 1 confers a substantially higher risk of developing eczema, especially the type that begins early in infancy and persists into adulthood. (16)

I previously discussed the importance of filaggrin in developing a healthy skin barrier. In fact, one of the skin proteins coded on the epidermal differentiation complex region of chromosome 1 is filaggrin. Studies have shown that up to 56% of people with eczema or atopic dermatitis have a loss of function mutation in the filaggrin gene. One study showed that 9% of people of European descent carried loss-of-function gene variations that predispose them to eczema. (7) There is also another genetic predisposition causing mutations in the region that codes for a protein called hornerin. Further loss of function or null mutations are being discovered for the coding of the other S100 family of proteins involved in the making of the stratum corneum.

More recently, a mutation was found in the claudin-1 gene. (14) It seems logical to me that these mutations could also exist in areas that code for keratin and collagen too. We have yet to discover all the mutations involved.

Mutations on any of these genes strongly predispose individuals to the development of eczema. (16) Loss of filaggrin function alone results in the inability to produce an effective barrier function of the skin, causing excessive drying as water evaporates too quickly from the epidermis, leading to itching, resulting in mechanical damage from scratching. This allows other irritants to enter the skin and cause further irritation and dryness, deteriorating the already weakened skin barrier and setting off a cascade of immune responses. (9)

Now recall when I discussed the formation of the healthy upper layer of the skin, the epidermis. The upper epidermis contains profilaggrin, a protein in the granulosum layer's granules. I mentioned previously how profilaggrin was incorporated into filaggrin. Filaggrin is an essential protein in forming the epidermal barrier as it binds to and aggregates the keratin, which gives hardness to the outer skin layer (3, 16); it is vital for skin cells to mature. Without filaggrin, the cells cannot collapse into the tough, flat corneocytes that form the outermost protective layer of skin, known as the cornified cell envelope. The cornified cell envelope is created as a direct result of filaggrin binding. These dead skin cells form the outer layer of our skin. (3, 9) Secondly, the filaggrin that remains in the cells helps to create the natural moisturising element of the skin. The lipids (fats) previously contained in the cell surround the corneocytes and keep them waterproof and supple. The water held by the histidine is released into the spaces of the epidermal cells, keeping the skin moist. This layer of water and fats is the natural moisturising factor, pivotal in keeping the skin healthy, moist, supple, and protected from external irritants.

Therefore, a filaggrin deficiency leads to dry, itchy skin, a precursor to eczema and is strongly linked to atopic eczema. At least 20 loss of function mutations have been identified to cause filaggrin deficiency. Not everyone with a single filaggrin gene mutation will have eczema or dry skin, and not everyone with eczema has a filaggrin mutation. It is estimated that 56% of eczema sufferers have a filaggrin gene mutation. However, as filaggrin is not the only protein coded for in the epidermal differentiation complex region, as more mutations are discovered, the percentage of people with loss of function mutations in other S100 proteins affecting skin production is expected to increase. (9) Hornerin is also expressed in the epidermis in the same location as profilaggrin and shows up in the stratum corneum. This would suggest that filaggrin and hornerin have similar functions. A study showed evidence that hornerin is also a component of the cornified cell envelope and that reduced expression of hornerin in the epidermis of patients with atopic dermatitis may also contribute to epidermal barrier defects. (14) As a side note, filaggrin deficiency is also associated with keratosis pilaris, which appears as tiny, hard, pin-sized, skin-coloured lumps on the upper outer arms and sometimes on the cheeks and legs. (9) Therefore, keratosis pilaris further indicates a possible filaggrin deficiency and gene mutation.

Inheriting more than one gene mutation predisposes individuals to eczema, particularly if they live in a westernised industrial area. Around 10% of people in the United Kingdom are said to have inherited a faulty gene copy encoding filaggrin, which results in reduced filaggrin levels in the skin. These are loss of function mutations; however, many different genes can have this loss of function mutation, not just one. Possessing a loss of function mutation results in an approximately 50% reduction in the filaggrin content in the skin. This loss of filaggrin affects people differently, from slightly dry skin to severely dry skin and cracked palms and feet. Inheriting more than one loss of function mutation proportionately increases the risk of developing atopic eczema, and if it does develop, it is often severe and persists into adult life. There is also a risk of developing severe asthma in individuals with these loss-of-function mutations. (9) In 2017, researchers tested the expression of the filaggrin genes present in the umbilical cords of newborn infants. The association between the loss-of-function mutations for producing filaggrin and subsequent eczema development was so strong they could predict with high accuracy which infants would develop eczema by three months of age. (10)

Researchers found two mutations in the KIF3A gene in another study, which encodes the protein kinesin. These mutations were confirmed to play direct roles in the development of eczema through a series of experiments in children. Loss-of-function mutations of this gene are linked to increased water loss through the skin, the development of dry skin, and the consequent damage that comes from scratching. Proper functioning of the KIF3A gene is essential because it helps cells to form primary cilia, which are bristle-like structures on the cell surface. They act as antennas to receive important signal information from other cells and use this information to help regulate water loss from the skin. Previous studies led by experts at Cincinnati Children's Hospital and others have shown that malfunctioning KIF3A in various body parts can predispose children to disease development. For example, in the skin, it can cause eczema; in the lung tissue, it can lead to asthma; malfunctions of the same gene in gut tissues can increase the risk of food allergies. (34) Thus, it is highly likely that mutations in this gene are involved in the development of the Allergic March.

The skin of atopic patients also contains significantly decreased expression levels of claudin 1. Claudin 1 is a protein that is encoded by the gene CLDN1. Claudins are necessary to produce the tight junction complexes that regulate the skin cells' permeability (how easy it is for water and molecules to pass in and out). While some claudin family members play essential roles in forming impermeable or impenetrable barriers to keep unwanted invaders out, others help to regulate the permeability of cells to substances that need to pass in, such as ions (electrolytes) and small molecules. Often, several claudin family members are expressed in relation to each other and interact with each other, which determines the overall permeability of the skin as a unit. Reduced claudin-1 also appears to be related to an increased risk of infection by herpes virus type 1 in those who suffer from atopic dermatitis. (40)

In 2002, two scientists, Tsukita and Furuse, published research showing that claudin-1 deficiency in mice led to higher-than-normal water loss from the skin and liver abnormalities, culminating in death. These animals showed no structural abnormalities but significant loss of function of the skin barrier. A similar clinical condition of claudin-1

deficiency was described in human infants as a disease called ichthyosis-
-sclerosis-cholangitis syndrome. (39)

I have already discussed how profilaggrin is 'carried' within the keratin granules, called keratohyalin. Cells should fill with keratin by the time they reach the skin's surface, where they collapse due to the action of the protease enzymes on the profilaggrin. (1) If there is a loss of function mutation in the gene encoding the keratin protein, this will also detrimentally affect the ability of cells to carry profilaggrin and histidine, and consequently their ability to become hard and cornified, and to carry sufficient water through the layers.

It stands to reason from what we have covered so far that any mutations in the genes encoding epidermal structural proteins such as filaggrin, hornerin, claudin-1, keratin, collagen, and kinesin, will cause the skin barrier to become defective, creating dry, itchy skin, which is then easily aggravated by scratching and easily infiltrated by pathogens and allergens. Put simply; your body does not have the building blocks it needs to create an effective skin barrier. This allows antigens to enter the skin and creates a cascade of responses that shapes how the immune system will respond to any future exposure to those antigens. (16)

As a side note, in a subset of older female patients who develop eczema later in life, an association with a mutation in the gene region coding for a substance called manganese superoxide dismutase has been observed. It is one of the most important antioxidant enzymes within the skin (15) and is generally produced in our body from food sources such as curcumin, broccoli, cabbage, and cruciferous vegetables. If you are female and have developed eczema later in life, consider the possibility that you could be deficient in this antioxidant and adjust your diet to incorporate more food sources. Even if you are not deficient, it is highly unlikely that increasing your intake of these will be harmful to your health. I have never heard of anyone dying from an overdose of vegetables. It is far more probable that we develop many diseases from a deficiency in vegetables.

In the chapter "Ditching the Itch", I previously described how histidine supplementation could support the body in producing a more robust and effective skin barrier. Now we can understand why. The amino acid L-histidine is rapidly incorporated into profilaggrin (healthy skin has a remarkably high histidine content of around 10%), and as it is hydroscopic (meaning it attracts water), it captures water and retains it in the cells, carrying it up through the layers of the skin. When the enzyme action occurs to collapse the cells, a process called proteolysis breaks down the proteins releasing the L-Histidine back into the skin as a critical moisturising component. (1)

L-histidine is a simple nutritional supplementation to find. Studies show oral supplementation with 4 grams of L-histidine dissolved in a morning fruit juice, once daily, for four weeks, significantly increased the filaggrin ratio in eczema patients by around 40% with a subsequent increase in barrier function and reduction in eczema severity and activity. This is a significant improvement and of a similar effect to mid-potency topical corticosteroids but with NO ADVERSE SIDE EFFECTS. The improvements even persisted for several weeks after supplementation ceased. (1) The scientists declared that L-histidine is a safe, convenient, non-steroidal intervention suitable for long-term use in managing atopic dermatitis, particularly in children. A word of warning though, L-histidine tastes quite bitter, so you either need something to hide the flavour when you take it or buy yourself some empty capsules to make your own supplements. You can purchase histidine already in capsule form, but they are only 500 mg each, so taking eight capsules a day to get to 4 grams will work out rather expensive compared to purchasing a bag of loose powder. There will also be other fillers and ingredients in the ready-made capsules that you do not need to take.

Additional studies injected L-histidine into rats to assess its effectiveness in improving skin barrier function. Researchers witnessed its incorporation rapidly (within 1-2 hours) into the profilaggrin within the keratohyalin granules. One-to-seven days later, it was subsequently released as free amino acids in the natural moisturising factor in the upper skin layer, the stratum corneum. This is a very rapid result. There is a direct association between reduced stratum corneum levels of free natural moisturising factor amino acids (including histidine and its antibacterial compound, urocanic acid) and the severity of atopic dermatitis (eczema). (1, 14) Furthermore, as the trials above both showed no adverse side effects with histidine supplementation for eczema patients, why is histidine supplementation not recommended as one of the first protocols to follow in treating eczema? It would certainly fit the Hippocratic oath of medical professionals that they will strive to "do no harm." Why was this not shouted from the rooftops and published in all the newspapers when it was discovered? Probably because there is no profit to be made from it. You cannot patent an amino acid, so you cannot hike the price up and make billions of dollars by promoting it. Meanwhile, millions of people continue to suffer needlessly because they are left unaware that this protocol even exists, let alone that it has been proven safe and effective.

In contrast, how many of the pharmaceutical medicines prescribed to treat eczema can claim to have no adverse side effects? Erm...I currently do not know of any.

So why do supplements work? They work because YOUR HEALTH IS NOT DICTATED BY YOUR DNA. That may be opposite to everything you have heard before, but we now know that epigenetic factors are far more powerful than DNA in determining a person's disease state. Epigenetic factors are your diet, lifestyle, exposure to environmental pollutants, and your mindset. In other words, just because your DNA contains a code that predisposes you to develop a specific disease, that code does not have to be turned on. Let us look at how epigenetic factors affect our health.

Right from the beginning of life, when a baby forms in the womb, cell division occurs, and portions of DNA code are activated to determine what happens next. The cells communicate through electronic signals produced within the cells. These signals are then converted to chemical signals, which convey the 'messages' between the cells. They develop into their respective body parts depending on the 'messages' communicated. If some of the cells are removed, even if they are kept alive and healthy, they stop developing. This shows that although the cells contain the DNA instructions needed to develop, it is their environment that determines whether the activation of these codes occurs. They need the communication signals from the other cells. This phenomenon is not limited to cell replication in the womb; it exists for the rest of life. Our cellular communication and the proteins our cells produce directly impact other cells and how they function. Therefore, it is the epigenetic factors determining the which, how, and when of our gene expression, not the DNA code in isolation.

I have recently finished reading an excellent book by Dr Caroline Leaf, a communication pathologist and audiologist with many decades of experience working in the field of cognitive neuroscience. She has pioneered much research on neuroplasticity (how the brain can remodel itself) and presents her findings in her book "*Switch on Your Brain.*" Dr Leaf clearly shows that mindset is fundamental to health, as our thought life directly affects our health via epigenetics. Our brains are physically changed by our thoughts, which can be evidenced by brain scans. Every thought causes the production of proteins that impact our memories, our perception of events, our outlook, and ultimately the gene expression of cells influenced by those proteins. She shares numerous studies showing incredible changes in the brains of people who had consciously changed their thought patterns and created new ones. These changes allowed them to change not only their ingrained subconscious belief patterns but also their health and wellness, as the proteins produced by the brain affect the function of other cells in the body.

The blurb on the back of her book begins with the statement, "You Are Not a Victim of Your Biology!" This is a crucial statement for eczema patients to grasp and backs up what I stated earlier: your DNA does not dictate your health. Ultimately, you must address your belief about eczema first if you desire to be healed. Eczema patients are so pumped full of statements like "eczema is incurable" by all the supposed experts that you can easily lose hope and start *expecting* treatments to fail. We will then find reasons to justify our beliefs, backing up our unwillingness to try new options with statements such as "I have already tried everything", or "it runs in my family, so I just have to learn to live with it", or "there is no hope for me." However, these beliefs, whether conscious or unconscious, will create proteins and the more you repeat them, the more those proteins will establish and entrench those beliefs. Tony Robbins has a highly effective technique for dealing with limiting beliefs. He likens any belief to a tabletop with the reasons used to justify it as the supporting legs. To collapse the table (the wrong belief), he asserts that you must remove the legs. Just as a table cannot stand up without legs, neither can a belief stand up if its supporting legs are removed. Therefore, regarding eczema, let us quickly look at the legs supporting the belief that you cannot be healed.

Is eczema really incurable? The internet is awash with testimonies from people who HAVE been healed. However, please remember that eczema is only a label. It is not what is wrong with you. You cannot be healed from a label, but you can find out what put you under that label in the first place and seek to resolve it. So, if people tell you eczema is incurable, just remind yourself that although they say the eczema LABEL is incurable, with a bit of detective work, the causes of eczema are discoverable, and THEY are curable. If it were not so, there would be no healing testimonials online, whereas there are many. We can therefore remove this table leg as it cannot stand up under scrutiny.

What about the statement I hear so frequently, "I have already tried everything!" Honestly? Have you really tried every single protocol in the entire world? I sincerely doubt it. I know for a fact that you have not yet implemented the things I reveal in the eczema spider; otherwise, you would not be reading this book. Therefore, we can safely remove that leg from the table too.

"It runs in my family, so I have to learn to live with it" is another one I hear, especially in the case of atopic dermatitis. I have already addressed this. You just learnt that your DNA does not control your health, and neither are you a victim of your biology. Your genes can be switched on or off depending on the environment of your cells and the proteins you create with your thoughts. Now we have removed the third leg of the 'eczema is incurable' table. I don't know about you, but I have not seen any four-legged tables that could remain standing with three of the legs removed. But to ensure the table entirely collapses, let me remove the final leg: "There is no hope for me."

Listen to me. As long as you are breathing, there is hope. As long as you have your free will to exercise your own health advocacy, there is hope. As long as you have your mental faculties intact to assess the latest information that comes to you, there is hope. So, with this table having no legs to stand on, please put aside all thoughts that you are wasting your time or that your efforts are hopeless. Instead, build a new table. Let us create a new belief: "My body has the ability to regenerate." Can we put legs under it to support it? Yes, we can. Leg number one is: "The internet has thousands of testimonies of people who have taken responsibility for their health and healed themselves by changing their lifestyles." Leg number two is: "There are still many therapies I have not tried because I have not even heard about them yet, so I have exciting opportunities to learn." Leg number three is: "I can influence my epigenetic environment and change my gene expression. I just need to learn how." And finally, leg number four is: "I have renewed hope because I am still here, I am still breathing, and I still have the capability to learn." Do you feel more hopeful for your journey now?

Consider other blocking beliefs you have held about eczema and write them down. Then, go through this technique again, disable the legs on those tables, and create new ones. This process literally rewires the brain, and although you may catch yourself thinking the old thoughts, you have created new ones; you can capture your old thoughts and consciously choose to replace them with the new ones. The more you think the new thoughts, the more proteins you make to establish those beliefs. The less you think about the old limiting beliefs, and the more you reject them as no longer relevant when they come to mind, the more your brain activity breaks them down until they no longer exist. As Dr Caroline Leaf states, you can literally be your own neurosurgeon and rewire your brain.

A new field of research called nutrigenomics is another branch of epigenetic studies. It reveals the interaction between nutrients and genes at a molecular level and how the bioactive compounds in certain foods can alter cellular signalling pathways. These can then regulate the expression of the genes responsible for producing inflammatory and anti-inflammatory cytokines. (22) I will address cytokines in Chapter 7 and the importance of nutrition in Chapter 10.

Disease states caused by epigenetic factors can cause the release of messenger RNAs that influence our DNA. They can even affect the germline (sperm and egg cells) and, consequently, our future offspring, hence the development of "inherited" diseases. However, there are amazing biomolecules called microRNAs which survive the digestive process. They are minuscule nano-sized particles secreted by all plant, animal, bacterial, and fungal cells and can regulate our gene expression by acting as silencers to messenger RNAs. As these silencer molecules can permanently reside within our germ cells, they can alter the genetic expression not just for us but also for our future generations. This has enormous implications. As scary as these messenger RNA molecules may sound (especially when they are now being used in 'vaccines' with unknown mid to long-term consequences), we now know that we can use micro-RNA molecules to our advantage by harnessing the power of the micro-RNAs in food to switch off disease codes. As these minuscule particles take up residence in our germ cells, they can override the gene codes for inherited diseases in our offspring. In simple terms, this confirms that although your DNA may contain the code for a disease or gene mutation, the microRNAs can silence the messenger molecules that would carry out the instructions of that code, effectively turning it off and saving you from the disease. (22)

This is an incredible discovery and a huge reason to eat more plants. However, there is one drawback; cooking and food preservation methods kill microRNAs. Therefore, if you are someone who finds eating raw plants as attractive as clawing your fingernails down a chalkboard, you will not be consuming these precious little 'keys' that can turn off your disease genes. This is just one reason why fresh fruits, salads, and veggie smoothies should be considered your best friends, not your enemies. Believe me; there are many more reasons too. Eating organic produce is also more beneficial to limit your exposure to the pesticides on food that may influence your gene expression. I have devoted a whole chapter to diet and nutrition so that we can dive deeply into this valuable topic.

We also need to limit our exposure to things that can cause our DNA to be damaged whilst in its unravelled state (there is always unravelled DNA somewhere in our body). For example, electromagnetic fields from cell phone towers and phones, radiation from microwaves and X-rays, toxic medications, and exposure to chemical pollutants in the air we breathe, the water we drink, and the products we use to clean our bodies, our homes, and our laundry all contribute to damaging our DNA. As we have learned, damage to DNA risks the development of mutations and susceptibility to numerous disease states.

Although we cannot leave the planet or wrap ourselves and our children up in impenetrable body suits to protect ourselves, there are simple, effective ways to limit your exposure. We have already addressed having water filtration systems installed in your home. I reiterate that these are extremely important. Municipal or urban water supplies are customarily treated with chlorine, and many have fluoride added despite the questions over its safety. Unfortunately, it can also be polluted with pesticides, heavy metals, lead from old deteriorating pipes, and estrogen hormones, especially in areas where sewage water is recycled. Women taking the estrogen contraceptive pill will pass estrogen into the water systems via their urine. In addition, industry and agriculture practices produce even more waste products that contaminate the water supplies with synthetic estrogens and chemical pollutants. The cleansing process of recycling sewage water or filtering water from natural water supplies is not sufficient to remove these estrogens. Estrogen contamination is already known to drastically reduce the reproductive capacity of fish, which has the potential to cause the collapse of entire fish populations; thus, it is no surprise that men's sperm counts are falling in areas where they are drinking estrogen-contaminated water. Unfortunately, with estrogen affecting the expression of certain genes, this excess synthetic estrogen has also been linked to the development of breast and testicular cancers and endometriosis. If you have not already purchased your water filters, please do so. Drinking contaminated water has far more implications for your health than eczema alone.

Using the hands-free on your mobile phone rather than holding it against your head or storing it in your bra, trouser pocket, or anywhere else close to your flesh (and genes) is a crucial protective measure. I now keep my cell phone in a Faraday bag. It blocks all EMF and 5G signals and also prevents any tracking ability or monitoring of private conversations. (Have you noticed that the adverts appearing on your phone are for the same topics you recently discussed whilst close to your phone?) This solution allows me to keep my phone with me for emergencies but limits my exposure to electromagnetic fields, prevents me from being tracked via my cellphone, blocks Artificial Intelligence from monitoring my private conversations and then targeting me with manipulative marketing adverts, and also allows me to control when I want to be contacted as my phone will only receive messages or calls when it is out of the Faraday Bag.

You do NOT want to live near a cell phone tower. They can lead to exposure to exceptionally high levels of electromagnetic fields, especially if they malfunction. I experienced this while living in a rented home in Trinidad. I had not noticed there was a mobile phone mast almost directly behind the property. Shortly after moving in, my entire family began to feel unwell, with varying symptoms. I was affected the worst because I spent most of my time in the kitchen at the back of the house. After much confusion and investigating trying to find the cause of our sickness, I finally spotted the mast through a small bathroom window. I was horrified that I had missed it, when viewing the home. However, being willing to give it the benefit of doubt, I purchased an EMF monitor to check if there was any cause for concern. To my dismay, there was only a single study area in the front of the house that was not registering on the monitor as having dangerously high EMF exposure. I promptly moved all my 4 children's beds into that small room and they all slept in that cramped space while I hurriedly looked for alternative accommodation. One of my neighbours on the street was a physicist at the local university and he took up the case of the EMF exposure. He discovered the tower was malfunctioning and exposing the entire row of houses to unsafe levels of EMF exposure! Thankfully, once we moved home, our health improved. Additionally, electromagnetic field exposure can also occur due to 'dirty wiring'. If you have yet to have the electric circuitry of your house checked or updated, I suggest you do so promptly. Old, inefficient wiring can not only be a safety concern from a fire risk point of view but also produce alarming levels of electromagnetic fields. All these sources of electromagnetic fields can have a direct impact on your DNA.

If you do have a cell tower nearby, or you wish to check the electromagnetic field exposure from wiring or electronic appliances such as microwaves, invest in an electromagnetic field monitor to check your exposure levels. Suppose the levels are high, and it is impossible to move home. In that case, you can take mitigating action, such as lining your windows with electromagnetic field-blocking curtains, painting the exterior walls with EMF blocking paint or wearing an electromagnetic field-negating necklace.

I reiterate, as previously discussed, you should be very mindful of the products you are putting on your body as many of them contain chemicals that are not helpful to your health. Many of these are known to be dangerous as they can interfere with proper hormone function (known as endocrine disruptors). A company called the Environmental Working Group regularly publishes lists of clean foods, cosmetics, and toiletries. I highly recommend making use of this resource. It may be annoying that we must make an extra effort to go hunting for safe products but let me remind you that your greatest power to influence the manufacturers is in your wallet. As consumers, we have the ability to influence what becomes a viable market or business opportunity. What we collectively buy less of will eventually stop being manufactured as it will no longer be profitable to produce, and what we demand more of will start to be produced more as there will be a growing market demand for it.

Bisphenol A in plastics is also a known endocrine disruptor. Therefore, it is far safer to store food and water in glass containers and limit your purchases of prepackaged foods stored in plastic containers. Other common exposures to plastic are drinking water bottles, plastic toothbrushes (you can purchase natural bristle ones), and plastic crockery or take-away containers.

Now that we have discussed the errors in the skin manufacturing process and the genetic mutations that contribute to them let us look at our eczema spider again. You have learned that genetic mutations can directly lead to excessively dry skin characterised by eczema.

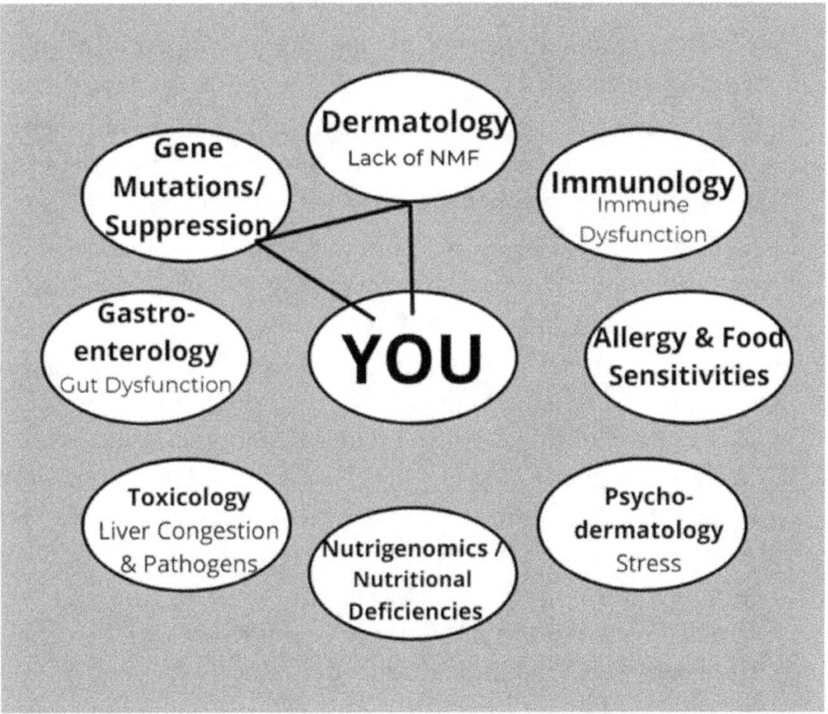

Next, we need to look deeper at what happens in the immune system when invaders and pathogens breach the skin barrier. This is where we start to see some fascinating loop systems developing that repeatedly drive the eczema response.

First though, let us review your action points for this chapter.

Action points

1. If you have not already done so, start filtering your water!

2. Supplement with L-histidine (4 g daily for adults), taken in a small amount of juice in the mornings.

3. Consider taking an organic amino acid supplement of all nine essential amino acids.

4. Start incorporating raw fruits and vegetables into your diet to provide yourself with microRNAs. Also, begin transitioning to an organic diet to limit your exposure to pesticides.

5. Consider purchasing or hiring an electromagnetic field monitor to locate sources of excessive electromagnetic field exposure in your home and work environment.

6. Stop carrying your cell phone against your body or holding it to your head when taking calls. Use the speaker or wire headphones instead. Bluetooth and wireless headphones are a source of electromagnetic field exposure to the head. Unless you need to be constantly contactable, consider using a Faraday bag for your portable electronic devices.

7. Start working towards using clean products on your body and face. Check the Environmental Working Group website for lists of safe, clean body care products and cosmetics. https://www.ewg.org

8. Start to transition to glass storage containers for your food items. It does not need to be an expensive venture. Jam jars and other glass containers can be washed out and recycled at home instead of discarded. This makes a cheap solution for healthier storage jars.

7

When You Don't Know JAK

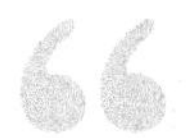

Contrary to popular opinion, inflammation is not always a bad thing."

Rollercoasters have been providing entertainment for adrenaline-hunting thrill seekers for many years. According to history.com, the first rollercoaster ride opened on June 16th, 1884, at Coney Island, Brooklyn, New York. Admittedly, that particular ride only travelled 6 miles per hour, so by today's standards, it would not be considered much of an adrenaline fix. In contrast, the fastest rollercoaster ride at the time of writing this book is the Formula Rossa in Ferrari World, Yas Island, United Arab Emirates. This ride reaches an astonishing top speed of over 149 miles per hour and generates a g-force of 1.7. Clearly, it is not one for the faint-hearted.

Rollercoasters were designed to complete a loop system, starting with a high ascent, which, once past the peak, creates sufficient kinetic energy as the car hurtles down the descending rails to propel the cars up the next incline. The system is repeated continually around the track until the brakes are applied at the end of the ride. Once the cycle is complete, the cars stop, and the participants can disembark, perhaps a little shaken but raring to go again, or maybe like me, feeling rather sick and vowing never to go on a ride like that again.

A rollercoaster ride provides an interesting analogy to the immune system, particularly the inflammatory cycles. Just as the ride is propelled by its own created energy until the cycle comes to a halt, inflammation is also driven by its own created energy systems, driving the inflammatory response to complete what should be a cycle, which then comes to a halt when healing has been achieved. It would cause severe problems if a rollercoaster ride did not stop when it reached the end of its cycle. Casualties and collateral damage would occur as a result. Similarly, when the inflammatory cycles get stuck and do not halt when they should, there are consequences, and damage ensues. In this chapter, we will look at what happens when the immune system gets stuck in the inflammatory cycle, as is often the case with chronic inflammatory conditions and autoimmune diseases.

We have already laid the groundwork regarding how the damaged skin barrier develops. Now it is time to peel the onion back further and look at what happens beneath the skin when someone develops eczema. It is here, below ground level, that the driving forces of eczema create loop systems that perpetuate the disease, much like a rollercoaster that does not stop, or as I mentioned earlier in the book, the strands of a spider's web that trap its innocent victim.

Do you remember I mentioned that *Staphylococcus* is a super-antigen because it causes a hyperimmune and inflammatory response? Well, I will now show you the inflammatory cycle that typically happens when *Staphylococcus* gets inside your skin. However, let me first explain the purpose of inflammation.

What is the Purpose of Inflammation?

The first thing you need to understand is that contrary to popular belief, inflammation is not always a bad thing. No, really, it is true. It is only when inflammation is chronic that it becomes detrimental to our health. Otherwise, inflammation serves a valuable purpose in healing our bodies. Let me explain further.

When we suffer from an infection or injury, we typically experience redness, swelling, pain, and irritation in an area. It may be in the nasal passages and throat if we are stricken with a viral infection such as seasonal influenza. Or it could be at the site of an injury if we have been involved in an accident. Certain cells in the immune system have a role in triggering the inflammatory response. These cells emit messengers called cytokines or chemokines that communicate to other cells to 'inform' them that an issue needs to be dealt with and assistance is required. They effectively recruit reinforcements to the site of the battle. One of the ways they do this is by releasing substances that cause the dilation of blood vessels in the vicinity of the infection or injury. This allows the flow of blood to the affected area to increase. Consequently, the site floods with extra immune forces, for example, cells that can fight invaders, cells that clear away other damaged cells or tissue, and other cells to make repairs where necessary.

When the issue has been resolved, different messenger molecules should be released with the help of other immune cells called regulatory T cells, or Tregs for short. These should calm and reset the immune system back to equilibrium and turn off the inflammation, or at least consistently turn it down as healing gradually takes place. Unfortunately, in the case of eczema, the immune system often gets 'stuck' in the inflammatory phase of the cycle because the skin never recovers sufficiently due to the cycles or loop systems that cause persistent, repeated flare-ups. This means that pathogens and irritants continue to enter the skin, repeatedly triggering the inflammatory immune response and suppressing the ability of Tregs to dampen the inflammatory response.

In this chapter, we will look at exactly how these cycles develop and what you can do to interrupt them naturally. Although the illustration seems complicated, it is actually quite fun to look at, especially as I have illustrated the main players using the characters from my book, **Superheroes Inside Me.**

Immune Cycle Dysfunction

The following picture shows the typical immune cycle that develops in someone with eczema. I promise it is not as hard to understand as it initially looks. Truthfully, there is even more going on than I can show in this drawing, but this is enough for you to gain an understanding of how the loop system develops.

As I have already covered the skin layers in detail, I have only drawn the ineffective final corneum layer and the bottom basal layer of skin here to save space. This is not as complicated as it looks if we go through the process step by step.

In step 1, you start with your damaged skin barrier function.

Then in step 2, some pathogenic bacterium such as *Staphylococcus* invade beneath the skin barrier.

In step 3, they disturb the keratinocytes and cause them to release a substance called thymic stromal lymphopoietin, often referred to as simply TSLP. (16) The thymic stromal lymphopoietin or TLSP pathway has been called the master switch for allergic inflammation because of the effects it exerts on numerous cells involved in skin inflammation. (29)

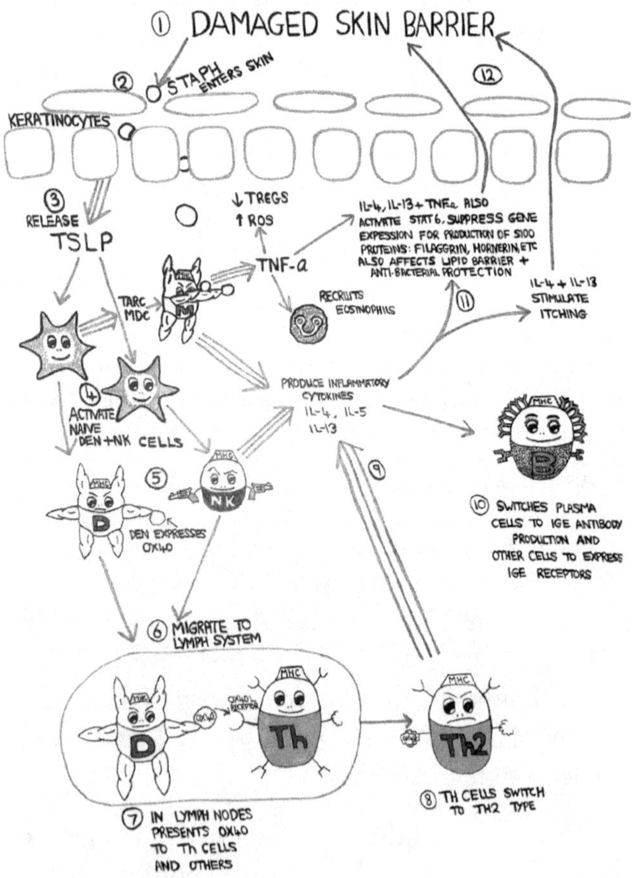

It is particularly produced by the keratinocyte cells when they react to the presence of *Staphylococcus* bacterium, which is one of the most common pathogenic invaders in eczema skin.

Thymic stromal lymphopoietin is a member of the cytokine family, one of those molecule messengers I spoke about earlier.

Step 4. One of the main effects of TSLP with regards to eczema development is the 'waking up' of both naïve dendritic immune cells and natural killer cells that reside in the skin and commissioning them into service as recruiters of immune re-enforcements.

The dendritic cells produce messenger molecules called chemokines. These are specific types of cytokines that attract other cells to the site of an invasion or infection. Two molecules of importance to our study are CCL17 (previously called TARC) and CCL 22 (previously named MDC). One of the effects of these inflammatory molecules is the recruitment of macrophages, a type of white blood cell I mentioned in the "Riddle of the Root" chapter (remember the big eaters I spoke about). Macrophages will always be involved in inflammation as they are the first responders of your cellular emergency services. They actively engulf and eat the invading pathogens that have infiltrated the skin. Macrophages are the primary producers of a substance called TNF-α (tumor necrosis factor-alpha). They also produce inflammatory cytokine messenger molecules called IL-4 and IL-13 (interleukins), which are particularly important in eczema, and which I will discuss more later. For now, we will focus on TNF-α.

TNF-α activates and recruits other immune cells called eosinophils, which are involved in inflammatory allergic responses (either increasing or regulating it depending on the situation). They also destroy cells that pathogens have invaded, kill parasite invasions, and fight bacterial invasions. You will typically find far more circulating eosinophils in the blood of allergic individuals than in those without allergies; the higher the number of allergies, the higher the level of circulating eosinophils. As they can increase the allergic response, having elevated numbers circulating can cause you to be more prone to allergic reactions and at more risk of severe allergic episodes.

TNF-α also kills cells that are becoming cancerous; therefore, it is in our best interest to have an expression level of TNF-α that enables it to do its job correctly. However, overly high levels of TNF-α are seen in many autoimmune diseases. For example, the inflamed joints of rheumatoid or psoriatic arthritis patients and those suffering from Crohn's disease, inflammatory bowel disease, and ulcerative colitis all display elevated TNF-α levels. This is not an exhaustive list. Do you remember in the chapter "Burdens Beyond the Boundaries" when I stated that eczema patients have a far increased risk of developing autoimmune diseases? One of the reasons for this is the persistently high levels of TNF-α produced by the macrophages as part of their immune response. It is highly inflammatory, and being such a small molecule, it can infiltrate tissue and cause inflammation and autoimmune issues. Studies have also shown that TNF-α is a major suppressor of the anti-inflammatory Treg cells that should keep the immune system calm. This would be logical, as, in times of inflammation, the body needs these cells to be suppressed to enable the inflammation to bring the necessary repair mechanisms to play. However, whereas in normal inflammation, TNF-α production would reduce as the issue or the damage is resolved, allowing the Tregs to start calming things down again, with chronic eczema (as with many other chronic autoimmune diseases), this does not happen. The constant production of TNF-α keeps the Tregs suppressed and the inflammation status running high. It is like the reset button has been disabled. (41)

A further issue caused by TNF-α is that it results in the long-lasting production of molecules called reactive oxygen species. Simply put, these are molecules that have missing electrons and, as such, have become unstable. As a result, they are harmful to the body as they can damage the lipids inside cells. (Remember, you need good quality lipids (fats) in your skin cells to help create an effective natural moisturising factor for the skin.) In addition, reactive oxygen species can also damage proteins that are essential to make the claudin for tight junctions, the histidine to carry water, the keratin for structural hardness, the collagen to bind or cement the skin cells, and so on. Furthermore, a build-up of reactive oxygen species can also damage your DNA and

RNA and interfere with cell signalling functions, which detrimentally affects the ability of cells to communicate with each other. (As I stated in Chapter 6, how the cells change and evolve depends on the cellular signals they receive from the other cells in their environment. Therefore, inhibiting these signal transduction pathways will affect the ability of your cells to function normally and healthily.) In addition, the claudin proteins are necessary for the cell signalling antennae, which regulate water evaporation from cells. Thus, disruption of claudin proteins will also detrimentally affect the ability of your skin to regulate its water loss.

These reactive oxygen species molecules have been shown to attract more helper T cells to the area, increasing the inflammatory reaction even further, as you will see shortly.

Step 5 is the thymic stromal lymphopoietin pathway causing the dendritic cells to express a molecule called OX40 and the natural killer cells to produce even more inflammatory cytokine messenger molecules, which include IL-4, IL-5, and IL-13.

In step 6, both the dendritic and natural killer cells start conducting their recruitment by leaving the skin and migrating to the lymph system (you can think of this as the underground metro system used by your cells to travel around the body), while continuing to send out their own molecule messengers.

In step 7, the helper T cells migrate to the lymph system to travel; TNF-a has summoned them. The dendritic cells will 'meet' them on their journey in the lymphatic system (think Metro station for your cells). When this happens, the dendritic cells present their OX40 molecules to the helper T cells for which they have the perfectly shaped receptors called OX40L. This OX40 molecule instructs them to differentiate or switch to become type 2 helper T cells, which occurs in step 8. Although I am showing the interactions between single cells, this process is happening within many cells. If you have eczema patches in multiple areas, it will co-occur in many places around the body. These interactions increase exponentially the more severe your eczema is.

Helper T cells are usually referred to as either Th1, Th2, or Th17, depending on the type of cytokine messengers they produce. Whether they become Th1 or the more inflammatory Th2 and Th17 types largely depends on the environment they are exposed to inside the body and what molecular messages they receive. It is the molecule messages that instruct the helper T cells to differentiate and become their different types.

What is the difference between Th1 and Th2 cells? According to Sergio Romagnani (126) in his article "T-cell subsets (Th1 versus Th2)", published on the Science Direct website, Th1 cells produce different cytokine messenger molecules to Th2 cells, namely IL-2 and TNF, whereas Th2 cells produce IL-4, IL-5, IL-6, IL-9, IL-10, and IL-13, which cause strong antibody responses from your other immune cells. They also cause an increase in the recruitment of eosinophils. It is a combination of both your environmental and genetic factors that determines whether your helper T cells polarise to Th1 or Th2. Atopic disorders in genetically susceptible individuals are said to be caused by allergen specific Th2 responses. (17) Th17 cells are also pro-inflammatory and produce other variations of cytokines. However, as neither Th1 nor Th17 cells seem to be particularly implicated in the eczema inflammation cycles, I will focus on what happens when the helper T cells switch to the Th2 type.

As shown in step 9, the Th2 cell begins to produce the inflammatory cytokines IL4, IL5, and IL13, known as interleukins. There are many different interleukins that carry varied messages and drive different reactions in the cells that receive them. They are given shortened names, such as IL and then a number. There are around 200 known cytokines, and 50 of these are drivers of disease. (37) I mentioned a few before when I was describing the differences between Th1 and Th2 cell types.

The ones we are particularly interested in from these Th2 cells are IL-4, IL-5, and IL-13, which all drive inflammation in eczema by recruiting more inflammatory cells to deal with the problem. The natural killer cells also produce the same inflammatory cytokines and drive the same responses. These cytokines cause three main events that drive the eczema flare cycle.

In step 10, the cytokines IL-4, IL5, and IL-13, released by both the Th2 and the natural killer cells, cause a particular group of immune cells called B cells (plasma cells typically involved in producing antibodies in response to infections) to change their antibody production and start to produce more IgE antibodies. These are the antibodies involved in allergic reactions. The same cytokines are also picked up by other circulating immune cells, which causes them to express IgE receptors when they did not previously do so. (16) Bearing in mind that your B cells have now been switched to produce IgE allergy antibodies, which will fit into those IgE receptors; you are building up the potential for an increasingly prevalent allergic nature. I will return to this in Chapter 8 when I explain the allergy cycles. For now, we will concentrate just on the inflammatory cycles.

Two more things happen in step 11 in response to the release of the cytokines IL-4 and IL-13. Firstly, they both produce itching. Yes, I know… like you did not already have enough. This has the knock-on-effect of causing you to scratch, which further damages the skin barrier and allows more pathogens to enter, and you start the thymic stromal lymphopoietin cycle all over again.

The second effect of these cytokines is the activation of the STAT 6 pathway within cells, which effectively means that a reaction occurs inside those cells, causing a molecule to travel to the nucleus (which is like the brain or engine room of the cell) and tells it to suppress or reduce the production of the S100 skin proteins, including filaggrin. Yes, the exact proteins you need to make more of to produce healthy new skin. Scientific studies have shown that increased levels of IL-4 and IL-13 significantly reduce the production of S100 proteins coded for within the epidermal differentiation complex on chromosome 1. (29)

An article published in 2017 titled "Feeding Filaggrin: Effects of L-Histidine Supplementation in Atopic Dermatitis" showed that although genetic mutations for filaggrin production and eczema are strongly linked, the situation is exacerbated further by the epigenetic effects exerted on the cells, which determines the disease severity. In addition, the actions caused by the inflammatory cytokines further reduce filaggrin processing and natural moisturising factor levels. These detrimentally impact the skin hydration levels and barrier integrity. (1)

Therefore, in addition to having possible gene mutations affecting your ability to produce adequate skin proteins, your cytokines are now suppressing the manufacturing of your skin proteins, which re-enforces the dryness, lack of natural moisturising factor, and ineffective barrier function that got you started on this cycle in the first place. Furthermore, even for those who do not have a genetic mutation, another study published in May 2013 stated: "It has also been demonstrated that Th2 cytokines such as IL-4 inhibit the expression of filaggrin and S100 proteins, thus impairing epidermal barrier, even in those WITHOUT genetic mutations for the coding of these proteins." (16).

This takes you to step 12, where you produce an ineffective skin barrier, which brings you back to step 1, where the rollercoaster ride begins all over again. Now you can see why you are so frustrated by repeated flare-ups and feeling like you are going around in circles. You are! But this is only one of the cycles. When we delve further into the workings of eczema, I will show you more.

Here are some more extracts from scientific documents confirming this information.

Worldallergy.org published a study, which was updated in May 2013, titled "Eczema: Pathophysiology." This is an excellent study that I highly recommend reading. It states that in addition to showing genetic mutations that predispose individuals to eczema development, having a dominance of Th2 cells producing cytokines such as IL-4 suppresses the expression of filaggrin and S100 proteins, which further impairs the ability to make an effective epidermal barrier. It went on to say that various studies have identified contributing factors to the mechanisms of eczema and that having Th2-mediated immune dysfunction plays a pivotal role in eczema development. The study also said that Th2 dominance occurs not just in the skin but also in the circulation, especially for atopic eczema.

Furthermore, the study details that the Th2 cells in the skin trigger an inflammatory reaction involving mast cells and eosinophil granulocytes (which I will cover more in the next chapter, Arresting the Allergic March). It is also the action of the Th2 cells secreting IL-4, IL-5, and IL-13 cytokines, suppressing the innate immune response of skin cells and causing lower amounts of antimicrobial peptides in the skin. This reduced innate immune response explains why the skin of eczema patients is frequently colonised with *Staphylococcus aureus*. The scientists in this study also demonstrated a direct correlation between the severity of a patient's eczema and the number of *Staphylococcus* bacterium resident on the skin. They stated that this is likely due to the *Staphylococcus* releasing toxins such as enterotoxin A or enterotoxin B into the skin. (16)

Another study published in 2011 stated, "A key protein in the formation of healthy skin is claudin-1 (CLDN-1), which has been shown to be deficient in eczema patients. It is inversely correlated with circulating eosinophil counts and serum IgE levels. These are markers of Th2 polarity and are a characteristic feature of atopic dermatitis patients… TNF-α inhibits… protein expression, directly affecting the epidermal barrier integrity." (29) This again confirms that the production of skin proteins is detrimentally affected by the cascade of events triggered by a Th2-dominated immune response.

A study published in 2016 titled "Skin barrier in atopic dermatitis: beyond filaggrin" showed that IL- 4 and IL-13 led to the decreased expression of filaggrin in the keratinocyte skin cells. It also reported reduced natural moisturising factor in the stratum corneum of individuals who suffered from eczema and those with mutations in their genes for filaggrin production. Changes in the skin barrier that occurred due to the filaggrin deficiency were seen to lead to inflammation and a reduction in the protein expression in keratinocytes. (39)

Therefore, the question must be asked: How can we break free from these inflammatory cycles?

JAK-STAT Inhibitors and Immunological Interventions

One course of action that has been used to treat persistent eczema is to use pharmaceutical drugs to target what is known as the JAK-STAT pathways that are involved in the inflammatory cycles. I previously mentioned a particular cellular pathway called STAT6, which is activated by cytokines and causes a tiny molecule to enter the cell's nucleus and influence the expression of genes within the cell's DNA. This causes the affected cells to produce their own cytokine molecules, which then recruit other cells into the inflammatory process, which keeps driving the inflammatory cycles.

The JAK-STAT pathways, particularly those activated by the IL-4 and IL-13 cytokine molecules, play a pivotal role in the chain of events leading to the development and persistence of eczema. They are involved in driving Th2 dominance, activating eosinophils, and suppressing the anti-inflammatory Tregs. (40)

Scientists have spent many years of research trying to develop pharmaceutical interventions to circumvent or disrupt these JAK-STAT pathways and, by doing so, interrupt the inflammatory cycle. In theory, it sounds like a great idea; however, the immune system is highly complex and attempts to interrupt its processes can cause unexpected side effects. At the time of writing this, the Food and Drug Administration has announced a delay in approving Incyte's Ruxolitinib cream, which has been marketed as an effective treatment for atopic dermatitis. This is also a JAK inhibitor that targets TNF-α. The theory is that reducing TNF-α can circumvent the inflammatory processes, reducing the severity of autoimmune conditions. The Food and Drug Administration delay has been caused by emerging concerns that interfering with TNF-α can result in an increased risk of heart inflammation and cancers. (111) I repeat, the immune system is highly complex. Sadly, we often only see the results of our interference once we are some way down the road.

In a publication called *Infectious Diseases in Children,* Douglas Kress, MD, a pediatric dermatologist at the University of Pittsburgh Medical

Centre Children's Hospital, stated: "What I am hearing is that in high doses, JAK inhibitors seem to be very effective, but they have a lot of side effects like suppressing the immune system, affecting white and red blood cell counts and liver function." Kress stated that these drugs seemed much safer at low doses but were much less effective. (33) If these drugs are not viable, what other treatments are available?

A relatively new pharmaceutical intervention on the market is immunological drugs that seek to disrupt the inflammatory cytokine cycles involved in eczema. One that is gaining in popularity is KY1005, commonly known as Dupixent. It is a fully human monoclonal antibody, which in simple terms, means that it is a genetically engineered human molecule designed to bind to the particular receptor I spoke about previously on the T cells called OX40L. Blocking these receptors with artificial molecules prevents the OX40 molecule expressed on the activated dendritic cells from binding to the receptor. The idea is that by blocking the T cells from interacting with the OX40 molecule, the processes that would have occurred within the cells to drive the inflammatory cycle will be interrupted. As a result, the cells will be prevented from differentiating into the inflammatory Th2 type. Ultimately, by blocking the interaction between OX40 and its target OX40L receptors, KY1005 is said to have the potential to bring the immune system back into balance by both suppressing the production of pro-inflammatory Th2 cells and maintaining the production of anti-inflammatory regulatory T cells. The idea is to reduce the number of TH2 cells in circulation and, consequently, the level of inflammatory cytokines they produce. This would theoretically allow Treg production to be increased. (36)

Eczema support groups have frequently posted questions and comments about Dupixent, asking for the opinions of those who have tried it. The responses of people vary. Some people speak of it almost as a lifesaver in giving them respite from the torment of their condition. Other people have tried it and suffered side effects that made it impossible to continue their treatment. The Dupixent website (Dupixent.com) lists the common side effects: eye and eyelid inflammation, including redness, swelling, itching, and cold sores in the mouth and on the lips.

They also list more severe side effects such as allergic reactions and anaphylaxis; fever; general ill feeling; swollen lymph nodes; swelling of the face, lips, and tongue; hives; itching; fainting, dizziness, and feeling light-headed due to low blood pressure; joint pain; and skin rashes.

As I have previously mentioned, we are all individuals, so our reaction to medications is also individual. When my children were on pharmaceutical interventions for their eczema, my family doctor told me that concerning prescribed medicines, "one man's cure is another man's poison" and that "trial and error are his only courses of action to determine the best therapeutics." Personally, and this is purely my opinion, I would rather exhaust all efforts to correct the internal issues naturally before I interfere with the workings of my own or my children's immune systems. Particularly concerning children, we are still at a very early stage in determining the long-term side effects of suppressing the body's inflammatory cycles. We have already established that inflammation serves a purpose. We do not want it to be switched off; we want it to be balanced and bought back to equilibrium, preferably without using anything that may give us other side effects to worry about.

There is also the issue of considering how long you want to take these medications. At roughly $37,000 USD per year (in 2021), if you do not have medical insurance covering or subsidising the cost (or a National Health Service as we do in the United Kingdom), then the expense will quickly become prohibitive.

Suppose you decide to stop taking Dupixent (or any other long-term eczema medication such as doxycycline antibiotics or steroids) for reasons of side effects or cost. In that case, you need to be aware that you may experience withdrawal reactions. Typically, the monoclonal antibody molecules of Dupixent block the OX40L receptors for approximately two weeks, which is why the medication needs to be injected bi-weekly. If you discontinue the treatment, the receptors will open again after two weeks. In theory, because of the interruption of the Th2 cycle, there should be fewer inflammatory cytokines in circulation. However, unless you have experienced healing to miraculous proportions and now have a restored skin barrier, the thymic stromal lymphopoietin cycle will still be running. This means that the keratinocytes are still producing the thymic stromal lymphopoietin, which wakes up the dendritic cells, causing them to make inflammatory chemokine recruiters and present the OX40 molecules on their surfaces. Thus, as the Dupixent wears off and the receptors open again, you could have a host of OX40-presenting dendritic cells just waiting for OX40L receptors to bind to. This will trigger a huge cascade of helper T cells flipping to the Th2 type, B cells switching to IgE production, and a flood of inflammatory cytokines being released again, including IL-4, IL-5, and IL-13.

I have personally worked with people who (against my advice) decided to suddenly stop taking their Dupixent medication without seeking medical guidance. As they did not gradually withdraw from the drug, they have unfortunately experienced this scenario. It caused them quite horrific withdrawal symptoms, which they stated were worse than their eczema had ever been, even before they started taking Dupixent. However, I have also heard from others who have tried Dupixent for a few months, did not like the way it affected them, and came off it with no withdrawal symptoms other than an end to the side effects they had been suffering. This reinforces the statement from my doctor that one man's cure is another man's poison. Not that immunological drugs are a cure in the real sense of the word; they are merely another symptom management system. They are, however, extremely profitable for the pharmaceutical companies selling them. Dupixent alone raked in over $5 billion (USD) in sales in 2021 (111), and they expected this revenue to increase by over 45% in 2022. This is only one eczema medication. Indeed, having chronic eczema patients to manufacture medicines for is highly lucrative.

I am not trying to demonise Dupixent or any other pharmaceutical intervention (despite being dismayed at the seeming profiteering). It is also not my intention to judge anyone who has, or is, using these treatments. Eczema can be so debilitating and tormenting; it can bring people to a state of utter desperation to find relief. If that is where you are, I have total compassion for you, and I hope that within the pages of this book, you will learn how to reset your body naturally and break the cycles that have held you trapped for so long. It would be wonderful if you could arrive at a place where you no longer need any medications as your skin is clear. It can happen. Eczema is not the incurable disease it has been made out to be. By actioning all the points, I am giving you, you can break the cycles by snipping the web strands that are feeding into each other and immortalising the disease state.

What can you do to correct immune dysfunction from a natural perspective? Firstly, please ensure you implement the measures I have already told you about in the previous chapters to minimise the external sources of irritation and dryness: taking amino acid supplements to give your body the support it needs, particularly histidine (adults 4 g a day) to create a more efficient skin barrier and natural moisturising factor, and also using topical probiotics to assist your skin's natural antibacterial protection. These help close the skin breaches that let the pathogens in and thus turn down the thymic stromal lymphopoietin cycle at the origin. In addition to these external methods, let me bring your attention to some scientific papers that address the internal inflammatory issues.

A very interesting experiment was published back in June 2014, where scientists tested the effectiveness of ginger in reducing inflammation in athletes. They found that strenuous exercise increased the levels of inflammatory cytokines in the blood, particularly IL-6 and TNF-α, which both illicit the effect of suppressing the innate immune system and leaving people more prone to infections. (23) TNF-α, as we have already discussed, also recruits more eosinophils, increasing the allergic potential and suppressing the Treg cells (which are responsible for calming your immune system). This is one reason why exercise can cause or exacerbate eczema flares. TNF-α suppresses the skin's innate immunity and leaves you more prone to overpopulation of pathogenic bacteria, further escalating the immune cycles I spoke of earlier.

The study concluded that 500 mg of ginger powder three times daily reduced macrophage activity and production of the inflammatory cytokines IL-6 and TNF-α. In fact, ginger supplementations were found to be even more effective than dual-action non-steroidal anti-inflammatory medications in reducing inflammation but with fewer harmful side effects. They also did not cause any unwanted interference with the actions of other antigen-presenting cells. How does ginger do this? The active compounds called gingerols and shogaols cause the immune modulating effects. In addition, they are highly effective prostaglandin inhibitors. Prostaglandins cause inflammation and are also largely responsible for painful menstruation cramps in women. Out of interest, I checked to see if there were documents assessing the effects of ginger supplements on reducing period pains, and I was correct. One interesting study conducted double-blind trials on women suffering from painful periods. The study showed that taking regular ginger supplements reduced both the level of pain and the duration of pain. However, ginger is a very safe treatment compared to non-steroidal anti-inflammatory medications, such as ibuprofen. It is a shame that women are not told about such a simple remedy by their doctors. This study not only shows how to minimise inflammation in eczema caused by exercising but also how ginger can be utilised to increase Treg production and short-circuit the inflammatory cycles without the side effects of pharmaceutical medications.

Ginger has been known to have medicinal uses for centuries and is one of the most well-known medicinal herbs. Search on Google Scholar or one of my favourite sites, GreenMedInfo.com. You will see hundreds of studies investigating and confirming the humble ginger plant's fantastic anti-inflammatory and healing properties, everything from suppressing inflammatory cytokines such as IL-4, IL-6, IL-13, and TNF-α (all involved in the eczema cycle), to protecting dopamine receptors in patients with Parkinson's disease, to anti-cancer actions and a whole host of other medicinal benefits that are too numerous to mention here. Therefore, including ginger in your diet is essential when embarking on any anti-inflammatory regime.

Ginger can be purchased in capsule form or used by grating the root into salads and stir-fries, adding chunks to your juicing recipes, and making homemade ginger tea (which is even more effective if you include turmeric and black pepper too). You can also add ginger to fermented recipes, for example, Kimchi or desserts and cookies (preferably sugar-free ones). Find ways to get ginger into your diet every day. Researchers have found that only 2 g daily of root ginger, either raw or boiled, elicits demonstrable anti-inflammatory effects in the body. (23)

The third way to hack your inflammatory response is to utilise probiotics, particularly those that contain *Lactobacillus rhamnosus*. Yes, this is the same one that was studied for topical application. Numerous scientific studies have shown that probiotics have many mechanisms by which they reduce inflammation, and they have been proven to reduce the Th2 dominance and help correct the Th1/Th2 balance. In addition, they also reduce inflammatory cytokine production and increase anti-inflammatory cytokines that help to reset the inflammatory cycles and recover equilibrium. (12,13,34,47) I will go into further detail about this in the chapter titled "The Rainforest Within." Your action points for this chapter are to add ginger into your diet every day and to start taking a high-strength probiotic that contains the *Lactobacillus Rhamnosus* strain; particularly one labelled Lcr35.

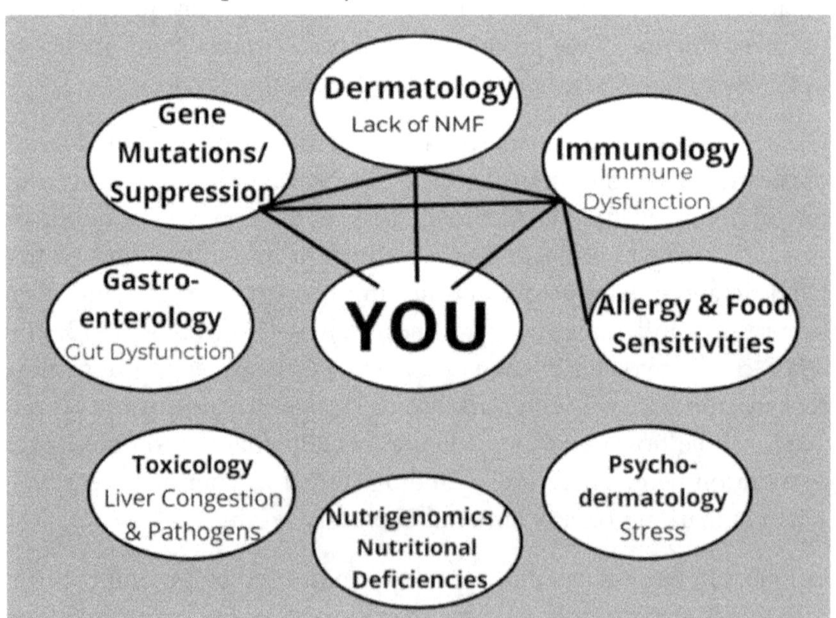

We have added more spider web strands, and we can now see the first cycle, how a lack of natural moisturising factor leads to a heightened immune response as the pathogenic bacterium invades through the damaged skin barrier. This, in turn, suppresses the expression of the genes coding to produce S100 skin proteins that are required to make a healthy skin barrier, thus perpetuating the problem of dry, itchy skin. It also flips your B cells to start producing IgE antibodies, which are involved in allergic reactions. Our next step is to examine what happens after this flip and how it leads to the Allergic March, creating yet another cycle to perpetuate the eczema flare and what you can do about it. Before that, though, here is your action point summary for this chapter.

Action points

1. Action the previous action point lists if you have yet to do so.
2. Add 500 mg of powdered ginger to your diet three times a day, or at least 2 g of fresh root ginger daily. This can be in the form of capsules; tea; raw in salads, juices, and smoothies; or cooked ginger in stews and stir-fries.
3. Start taking high-dose probiotics that contain 300–500 mg of Lactobacillus rhamnosus.

8

Arresting the Allergic March

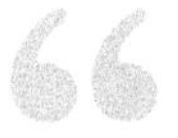

*The term 'friendly fire' is an oxymoron.
There is nothing friendly about being fired upon,
regardless of who is pulling the trigger."*

In every war, there is risk; the risk of losing the battle, the risk of collateral damage (innocent civilians being caught in the crossfire), the risk of retaliation against assets, and so much more. There is much to consider and debate regarding both the virtues of peacekeeping and the perils of outright war. This book is not the place for discussing the rights and wrongs of war, but there is one risk that is shared both by those involved in physical warfare and those battling chronic eczema, and in both cases, it can cause much damage. These are the circumstances that are termed 'friendly fire'. Let me tell you about the Cap Arcona incident to illustrate what I mean.

This tragic event occurred in the final days of World War 2 in Lubeck, Germany. The war was almost over. Thousands of allied war prisoners and over 4000 inmates from Nazi concentration camps were loaded, by Germans, onto three ships in Lubeck harbour. These passengers had survived untold horrors, and against all odds, when so many others had perished, they were still alive.

As the boats pulled out into the waters and began their journey, nine British Royal Air Force Typhoons flew into the area to conduct an anti-shipping strike. Apparently, the Scandinavian government had passed intelligence to the British to inform them of the prisoners of war and death camp surviving passengers. However, the information was not passed on to the local mission planners due to a severe communication breakdown. This meant those flying the Royal Air Force Typhoons were left to conduct their mission with incomplete or incorrect communication. Tragic and deadly consequences resulted.

Believing the German ships were filled with fugitive Nazis trying to escape to Scandinavia, they targeted all three ships, swooping low and unleashing a torrent of arsenal on them, sending the passengers into a fearful and quite justified panic. The Schutzstaffel (commonly known as SS) guards who were onboard decided to abandon the ships; however, before doing so, they fired into the terrified crowds, mowing down multitudes of their prisoners. German tugs and trawlers came out into the harbour to rescue some 400 of the SS guards from the freezing waters and burning ships, but they did not assist the prisoners. However, to the Royal Air Force pilots, seeing this German rescue attempt would have confirmed, in their minds, that the ships did indeed contain fugitive Nazis. Consequently, as the surviving prisoners made desperate attempts to escape by jumping from the burning vessels into the frigid waters and trying to swim to shore, the Royal Air Force pilots repeatedly flew in low, firing upon what they believed to be the fleeing enemies. Even those who mustered enough strength in their emaciated state to reach the shore were mercilessly shot in the water by the SS guards. In total, around 7000 prisoners of war and concentration camp prisoners perished either from the initial bombing, drowning, being shot in the water, or sinking in the ships. The Cap Arcona incident has been called the deadliest incident of 'friendly fire' in history. (56)

The term 'friendly fire' is an oxymoron. There is nothing friendly about being fired upon, regardless of who is pulling the trigger. But, unfortunately, it is all too common, and historical accounts of war are incomplete without the accounts of those killed by supposed 'friendly fire'.

Wikipedia describes the term 'friendly fire' as being caused primarily by either error of position, when fire aimed at enemy forces accidentally kills one's own forces, or by identification errors, where friendly or neutral troops are incorrectly identified as foes. The body is also capable of causing injury or death by identification errors, wrongly determining something as an enemy when it should be welcomed as an ally or tolerated as neutral. This misidentification is typical of the allergic response.

The information we examined in the previous chapter has laid the groundwork for understanding the Allergic March. You have already seen that having an overly dominant Th2 response causes a cascade of reactions that have triggered your B cells to switch to IgE antibody production. Now, we look at how having a defective skin barrier function allows allergens to enter the skin and trigger misidentification that is typical of allergic 'friendly fire'.

Consider, for a moment, how food and particles from the environment should generally enter our bodies. Do they go directly into our bloodstream from the outside world? No. They are usually ingested through our mouth and nose. What is the importance of this? Well, by entering the body through these channels, they will encounter our natural filters before they reach the blood supply. This allows our body to break them down into smaller constituent parts, as in the case of digestion, to sterilise them in our stomach acid, or to filter them through nasal hairs. Our tonsils also contain many white blood cells (immune cells, including macrophages), which can mount an immune response to invaders before they fully enter the body. In the case of viral infections, it may be contained in the throat; however, these immune cells may also travel to the lymph system to warn and prepare the rest of the immune cells. Consequently, they will be ready to fight effectively if the invasion spills over to other areas. This is also why those who have had their tonsils removed can be more susceptible to respiratory infections; their sentry-like first point of contact for potential pathogens has been removed, and consequently, their bodies have lost that ability to provide the early warning system to other immune cells.

Regarding food, we digest it as it passes through the gastrointestinal tract. By the time it is absorbed into the body, it is safely broken down into its nutrient parts and can be used effectively by the cells. Your blood cells are not supposed to encounter undigested or unfiltered particles of food and environmental proteins. However, this is precisely what happens when the skin layer is breached. Undigested food proteins and environmental allergens can pass through the broken skin barrier and encounter the immune cells in the dermis layer. The immune cells do not recognise these as the friendly or neutral particles they would be had they entered through the correct channels and wrongly identifies them as foes. Therefore, 'friendly fire' is triggered. For example, scientists have shown a significant relationship between having the type of eczema linked to filaggrin mutations and the resulting dry defective skin barrier, with the development of a peanut allergy that is driven by having IgE antibodies to peanuts. Allow me to show you, with another one of my course drawings, how this IgE response continues to drive the cycles of eczema flare-ups. (39)

To recap, we have already established that patients with atopic dermatitis exhibit changes in barrier function caused by deficiencies in skin proteins, decreased expression of filaggrin, and genetic mutations within the epidermal differentiation complex portion of chromosome 1, such as those resulting in loss of function mutations in skin protein codes. Scientists have long established that these mutations are known to increase the risk of developing eczema in infanthood, along with atopic issues such as asthma, allergies, elevated blood levels of IgE antibodies, and the type of atopic dermatitis that persists into adulthood. Their studies indicate that the increased skin permeability is causing greater exposure to allergens through the skin. (39) We have also seen that the Th2 dominance and resulting inflammatory cytokine milieu flips the plasma cells to IgE antibody factories. Thus, what happens after the B cells switch?

Please look carefully at the following picture.

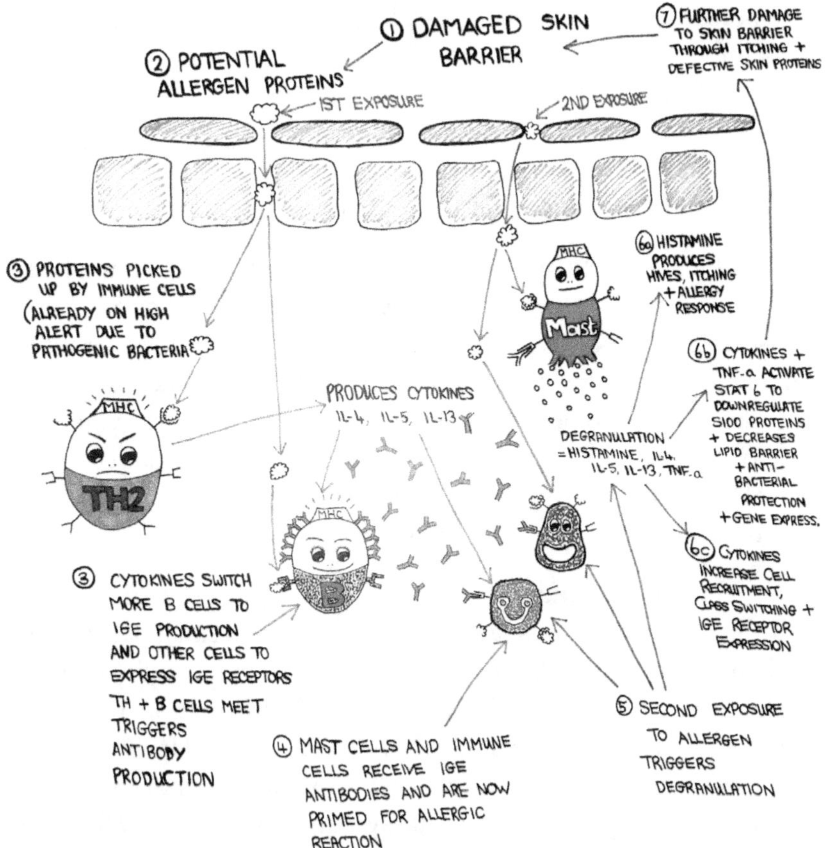

Just as pathogenic bacteria can breach the defective skin barrier, potential environmental allergens can also. This is step 1. Proteins are incredibly tiny, so small that they cannot be seen with the naked eye. This is why we can experience allergic reactions without us seeing any trace of the allergen. Therefore, we do not have to SEE a large dollop of allergenic food to experience an allergic response to its proteins.

In step 2, the allergens pass through the epidermal skin layer (remember it is only as thick as a sheet of paper) and encounter the dermal layer, where resident immune cells are already conducting inflammatory responses to deal with the pathogenic bacteria that have infiltrated your skin barrier. At some point, in your body tissues, both your Th2 cells and B cells (plasma cells) are going to encounter and 'destroy' what they perceive to be this new invading enemy, but which are those minute food proteins or environmental allergens such as pet dander, dust mite faeces, and pollen. (For the sake of our illustration, I will use peanuts as an example.) Your immune cells are already on high alert as they respond to the inflammatory cytokines being released due to pathogens entering your skin.

Your body is cleverly designed with many safety protocols in place to prevent mistakes. Unfortunately, however, they do still occur. One of these safety precautions is that just destroying an unknown or unrecognised particle in the blood is not sufficient to trigger the manufacture and release of antibodies to that potential invader. If it were, you would start to produce antibodies against yourself every time your cells killed one of your own rogue or decaying cells. This would obviously be very detrimental. Hence, the safety catch in step 3.

Your helper T cells and B cells are called antigen-presenting cells, as after they destroy an invader, they present or post small particles of it on their 'display boards', called the major histocompatibility complex. Antigen-presenting cells do this to 'share' information with other antigen cells about invaders they have encountered. Having multiple cells presenting the same antigen would indicate a more significant problem requiring greater immune system involvement. When your Th2 cells meet your B cells in the lymph system, they will recognise that they both have encountered the same enemy, as evidenced by the displays on their major histocompatibility complexes. This confirms a current 'invasion' and triggers the antibody release. Remember, from the last chapter, that the cytokines IL-4, IL-5, and IL-13 cause the class switching of B cells so that they produce the IgE allergy type of antibody. Now they will make the IgE antibodies to whatever the allergen was, in this case, peanuts. The antibodies will then spread out and attach to any other protein invaders with the same molecular structure, tagging them for destruction.

Now we get to step 4. Certain cells in your body have perfectly shaped receptors to receive the IgE antibodies. Mast cells are the primary ones involved in the eczema reaction; however, the inflammatory cytokines also signal to other cells, for example, eosinophils and basophils, to begin to express IgE receptors. The antibodies fit into these receptors, and these immune cells are now effectively primed and ready for an allergic response when they next encounter that allergen. (9) You do not experience an allergic reaction to the first exposure to a potential allergen. That initial exposure merely sets the stage and 'tells' your cells that the particular protein is to be seen as an allergen. The second exposure causes the allergic reaction, which is step 5.

The mast cells, eosinophils, and basophils all contain granules of histamine and other allergic mediators. The next time your immune cells encounter that allergen protein, they will react by a process called degranulation. This basically means that they release a burst of their granular contents to 'destroy' the invading protein. Their contents are very helpful for destroying parasites. If you consider that your body would 'expect' parasites, not food proteins, to invade through the skin, it makes sense that the allergic nature actually developed to attack parasites, not allergens. In addition, immune reactions can develop via a leaking gut, but this involves different antibodies, namely IgG.

Interestingly, IgG-producing cells are also involved in responding to parasite invasions through the gut lining, for example, from parasitic worms. Researchers have found that having parasite infections such as helminths and tapeworms increases the level of IgE responses in the body, both in IgE-producing cells and in cells expressing IgE receptors. This is another reason why I believe the allergic nature comes from the body thinking it is attacking parasites. In cases of genuine parasitic infections, it has been found that eczema patients can have allergic antibodies to the faeces of parasitic worms, which can also cause dermatitis-type rashes and itching.

Returning to our allergic flowchart, the unfortunate side effects of the histamine and other compounds being released when these cells degranulate are hives and itching. The action of degranulation also triggers the release of additional inflammatory cytokines, including IL-4, IL5, IL-13, and TNF-α, which continue to drive the allergic response by recruiting more immune cells to the area, re-enforcing the class switching of plasma B cells to produce IgE antibodies, and causing more immune cells to express the IgE receptors. (61) Therefore, this allergic response becomes an inner self-perpetuating cycle. To add further insult, they also activate the STAT6 pathway within the cells, which influences gene expression and the downregulation or suppression of the S100 skin proteins (such as keratin, filaggrin, hornerin etc.). This restricts your ability to generate a new healthy skin barrier, along with the lipid barrier and antibacterial protection, which leads to the final step in the circle. The cytokines also have the effect of inducing itching too, which we covered in the last chapter. This leads you to scratch and further damage your skin barrier.

In step 7, we have cycled back to having a damaged and dysfunctional skin barrier that is dry, itchy, compromised, and allows the entry of pathogens and potential allergens, triggering the release of more thymic stromal lymphopoietin from the disturbed keratinocytes. The rollercoaster fails to stop again, and off you go on another cycle.

Not all forms of eczema are associated with IgE, but atopic eczema does have a clear IgE antibody association and is characterised by increased levels of IgE antibodies circulating in the blood. (16) However, now that you understand how the breaches in your skin barrier lead to both these immune and allergy cycles, you can see why anyone with eczema has an increased risk of developing environmental and allergic sensitivities, regardless of which form of eczema they began with.

In fact, there is such a distinct allergic tendency in patients with eczema; it surprises and frustrates me that so many patients are told by their doctors that they (or their children) do not need allergy tests. Particularly in the case of infants, I frequently hear from their parents that physicians will not allergy test children under 12 months of age. Children with eczema should be tested for allergies as soon as physically possible. One of my daughters was only four months old when she was tested and confirmed to be allergic to many foods. I even stopped eating them myself to avoid minute proteins from my diet affecting her through my breast milk. Some allergists have told me that this is impossible as food eaten by the mother is digested and cannot possibly

---

trigger an allergic reaction via breast milk. I beg to differ with this opinion. I pinpointed nearly all my children's IgE allergies before they were even weaned. I did this by breastfeeding and keeping a food diary of everything I had eaten and how their skin looked. I saw clear patterns emerging. When I ate an offending food, their skin would flare with eczema 24 hours later. This could not have been caused by food proteins on my clothes, as the time taken to react to an IgE allergen would have been much more rapid if that were the case. In addition, I frequently changed my clothes, washed my face, and brushed my teeth after eating anything I suspected of being an allergy trigger to ensure my tracker was accurately recording reactions to my milk and not minute protein particles on me.

As the previous chapter shows, helper T cells play a significant role in regulating and switching IgE antibody production. Once helper T cells have differentiated into Th2 cells in your lymph system, they induce the plasma cells to switch to IgE antibody production through their cytokine production; this is a typical hallmark of atopic eczema. Sufferers then develop increased levels of both total and allergen-specific IgE antibodies in their blood as they embark unwittingly on the allergic cycle I have just described. These IgE antibodies are the ones that cause type 1 allergic reactions, the ones with a rapid allergic response, which are frequently tested for by skin prick tests. Skin prick tests utilise the allergic mechanism I just described to test for sensitivities. Pricking suspected allergens into the skin causes a disturbance of the underlying mast cells. If they have already been sensitised to those substances, degranulation will occur, with the resulting histamine release causing a hive to develop. The more histamine released, the larger the hive tends to be, allowing perceived sensitivity to be measured. However, false negatives and false positives can occur, so the results alone should not be relied upon as absolute truth. Some allergic priming can also occur in and around the gut rather than the skin, which is why some allergic reactions result in gastrointestinal symptoms rather than skin reactions. Blood tests are an excellent way to double-check the results and can provide a larger spectrum of results if tests for other antibodies are also conducted.

Allergic reactions to various foods are well known to exacerbate eczema in young children, which is why they should be allergy tested at the earliest opportunity. The most common allergens are milk, egg, peanut, soy, and cereals, including wheat. The Allergic March then ensues, and the number of allergies increases. Why does this happen? There are two main reasons. Firstly, the damaged skin barrier allows more environmental and food proteins to infiltrate the dermis layer and encounter the immune system. Secondly, there is a process called molecular mimicry or cross-reactivity at play.

In Chapter 6, I spoke about how proteins are like Lego structures made from individual bricks (amino acids) put together in sequences according to the instructions in the DNA code. When your cells recognise an invader as a threat and make antibodies against it, it is the protein part that they identify as the 'wanted criminal'. Proteins are made of sequences or chains of amino acids. One problem that can occur is that your cells can also react to other foods with a similar amino acid sequence. As you have already made antibodies to particular amino acid patterns in some foods, you will find yourself cross-reacting with other foods. This explains why people with allergies to cow's milk often also react to soya and goat's milk, or those with allergies to one form of nut quickly develop allergies to other nuts. It is a case of mistaken identity, which can progress rapidly because it bypasses the safety protocol that requires your B and helper T cells to have encountered the same invader. As far as your cells are concerned, those proteins look remarkably like those already identified as a foe, so they may be trying to sneak through the defences in disguise. Consequently, they give the command to open fire. As a result, the allergic arsenal is unleashed at ever more food and environmental triggers.

Although these IgE-mediated reactions are the most recognised ones, there are also non-IgE-mediated reactions to food and additives caused by hypersensitivities involving different antibodies or none at all. (16) Some food additives can worsen atopic eczema, but they may not show on a skin prick test that looks for IgE-mediated reactions or blood tests looking for delayed reactions. Some reactions involve IgM, IgA, and IgG antibodies, and IgG is even further categorised into IgG1,

IgG2, IgG3, and IgG4. These reactions are caused by insufficiently digested food particles entering the bloodstream via small leaks in the gut lining and being picked up by the immune cells in a similar way to what happens through the external skin barrier. The lining of the gut has the largest proportion of IgA and IgG antibody-producing cells in your body. These cells typically 'guard' your mucus-producing areas, such as your gut, nose, throat, and genitals. Most IgM-producing cells are found in your spleen; these are naïve B cells that have not yet been switched to produce other antibodies. Just as undigested food proteins trigger your plasma cells to produce IgE antibodies when they pass through the skin barrier, undigested proteins passing through the gut lining trigger production of IgG, IgA, and IgM antibodies. The same problem with cross-reactivity can occur here too. However, in this case, it is not only similar food proteins that are being mistakenly identified as a foe, but it can also be the proteins that make up your own body tissues. If you have ever wondered how people develop autoimmune diseases when our immune cells should know how to tolerate our own body, this is how. The antibodies released to 'identify' enemy protein structures mistakenly attach to body parts that are of a similar amino acid sequence, 'flagging' them for immune attack by your helper T cells. IgG antibodies are extremely small and so can pass into body tissues and accumulate there, causing the immune cells to attack those areas. IgG antibody accumulation has been seen in many sites of autoimmune inflammation. It explains why eczema sufferers have a significantly higher risk of developing other autoimmune diseases than people with healthy skin. The leaky gut allows antibody production against food, leading to cross-reactivity with other body tissues. Those of particular interest to eczema sufferers are the lectins from lentils and the agglutinin proteins from wheat, soybeans, peanuts, and beans. These all cross-react with proteins in the skin, causing antibodies to be made against your own skin proteins and flagging them for attack by your helper T cells. In addition, an alarming number of other organs and tissues in the body have been identified by scientists as being targeted by molecular mimicry from leaking guts, including the brain, causing neurodegenerative diseases and cognitive decline; the eyes, causing sight deterioration; the parietal cells of the pancreas, leading to diabetes; the thyroid gland, leading to Grave's disease and Hashimoto's disease; the cartilage, leading to arthritis; the myelin sheaths, leading to multiple sclerosis; the heart, leading to heart disease; and so many more including many cancers. (103) This is not something to be ignored. Do you remember what I said right at the beginning of the book: if you ignore your body when it is in dis-ease, it will cry even more loudly? This is why molecular mimicry leads to autoimmunity. These antibodies to self can be present in the body for up to 10 years before the autoimmune disease manifests itself. The good news is that you can switch this process off.

Antibodies have a half-life, much like radiation does. This means they deplete over time if no further exposures encourage their production. Therefore, if we completely avoid the foods we have discovered are causing our cells to release antibodies which cross-react with our own body tissues, the levels of those antibodies circulating in our bloodstream will reduce, and so will the inflammation caused by those antibodies. For this to work effectively, you should arrange testing with a Functional or Integrative medical professional who can help you ascertain, firstly, whether you have antibodies to self, and secondly, which foods are the sources of this cross reactivity. They will also be able to advise you regarding any other foods with a similar molecular structure that you should also avoid whilst you are reducing your antibody load. I experienced this phenomenon, albeit unintentionally when we moved to Trinidad. As I previously mentioned, one of my children had a high allergic sensitivity to Birch tree pollen and consequently developed Oral Allergy Syndrome. She started to manifest allergic symptoms to many raw fruits and vegetables. Her allergist advised me that this was just the path of the allergic march. However, after moving to Trinidad, where no Birch trees grow, her sensitivity to raw plant foods started to reduce. We have now lived here for six years, and she happily eats raw plant foods without experiencing any allergy symptoms.

Molecular mimicry also happened with one of my daughters, who developed a thyroid goitre at only nine years of age. It was caused by her doctor telling us she had to consume wheat for six weeks to facilitate her having a celiac test. This was despite my objections that she had already had a previous positive IgG blood test for wheat. However, he informed us that the National Health Service would no longer write her wheat-free bread and pasta prescriptions if we did not consent to the test. Feeling bullied into acquiescence, I allowed her to eat wheat for six weeks until she woke me early in the morning to complain that she could not swallow properly. When I switched the light on to check her throat, I was horrified to see a clear and prominent goitre in her neck. I took her to the doctor early that morning, and she immediately sent her to the hospital for tests and examinations. After ruling out thyroiditis and hyperthyroidism, the consultants finally admitted that it was likely due to the wheat consumption. I guess that could also be classed as another form of iatrogenesis: harm originating from my physician. Indeed, it should be considered medical malpractice for a doctor to instruct their patient to eat something for which they have a proven, blood-confirmed allergy. My daughter must now strictly avoid all wheat products and foods containing wheat as an ingredient, as she must ensure she does not trigger any further antibody production against her thyroid gland. If I had known then what I know now about molecular mimicry, I would have refused the celiac test and told them to stuff their wheat-free food prescription. Mothers are often bullied into ignoring their maternal instincts because we are not the experts. However, just because we might not have medical degrees does not mean we are not experts. When it comes to our own children, we ARE the experts. No one knows them more than we do. Parents, do not allow yourself to be pushed into accepting protocols that your gut instinct is telling you are wrong. Do your research and become the best advocate you can be for your family's health.

At the time of writing this book, scientific studies have linked wheat consumption to over 200 different medical conditions. (55) It is one of the food items we examine in greater detail later in the book. (In my previous family book, Superheroes Inside Me, you can also learn more about the interactions between your immune cells and molecular mimicry through fun stories.)

Exposure to some allergens considered to be airborne, such as house dust mites, cat dander, mould, or pollen, can also cause eczema flare-ups. (1,16)

However, when you see how allergies typically develop by the proteins entering the damaged skin barrier and triggering an immune response, you realise that eczema sensitisation to these airborne allergens can occur through the skin rather than the lungs. This is why I stated earlier in the book that I recommend eczema patients do NOT dry clothes outside on the clothesline during high pollen seasons. Minute amounts of pollen can become attached to the clothes and then enter the skin via the damaged skin barrier, thus sensitising the body to pollen. The same is true for dust mites, cat dander, and mould. Some clients I have worked with have tested positive for allergies to their furry friends, but re-homing their pets would be heartbreaking. In these cases, I advise people of simple methods to minimise their exposure to pet dander. Measures such as keeping pets out of bedrooms, using dust mite-proof covers over the beds or chairs their pets sit on, and air filtration devices significantly reduce allergen exposure. The dust mite covers are not primarily to keep dust mites out of the furniture, although that is an added benefit, but rather to protect the furniture from pet dander. It goes over the top of all the bedding, not directly on the mattress. This way, you can roll back the cover and retire to a dander-free bed, resulting in much better rest with reduced allergic symptoms.

Another type of 'friendly fire' or cross-reaction is when the immune system mistakenly identifies food proteins as airborne allergens due to the similarity of their protein particles. This leads to a condition called oral allergy syndrome, which one of my children developed. She was highly allergic to birch tree pollen but then developed intense oral irritation if she ate any raw fruits and vegetables with a similar protein structure to birch pollen. The list included apples, carrots, peaches, nectarines, plums, and cherries. She could eat them cooked (which changes the protein structure), but not raw. Oral allergy syndrome can cause alarming sensations in the mouth. However, in my daughter's case, she could remove the irritation quite quickly by either holding an antihistamine in her mouth or, once we learned of the power of vitamin C, by taking a high dose of vitamin C, which I will explain later in the chapter.

When we moved to Trinidad, where there are no birch trees, my daughter gradually regained the ability to eat these raw foods because antibodies do not live forever. They have a half-life, much like nuclear radiation, which is the time taken for the number of antibodies to reduce in half and start dying off. If no new ones are being made, the level of antibodies in the bloodstream reduces until the reactivity stops and the inflammatory cycle is reset. This is a crucial principle in healing from antibody-related inflammation.

There are also known skin irritants aside from the typical allergic triggers. Sensitivities can develop to chemicals in detergents, fragrances, air fresheners, and even rough or manufactured fabrics like wool or polyester. One lady told me she had been diagnosed with an allergy to leather and consequently could no longer wear any leather shoes or have any leather furniture in her house as it would cause her skin to flare with terrible eczema. Sometimes, these are genuine allergies to the material, but more often, they are reactions caused by the chemicals used in the manufacturing process or to treat the final product. We cover this more in Chapter 12.

Another allergy scientifically linked to eczema, but I have never heard of anyone being tested for it, is a somewhat controversial topic. In brief, a study conducted back in 1992 showed that the aluminium-based diphtheria-tetanus-pertussis (DTP) vaccine commonly given to infants at around eight weeks old is linked to the development of an aluminium allergy, which leads to eczema. Is it just a coincidence that infant eczema most commonly develops around eight weeks old, the same age as when the diphtheria-tetanus-pertussis vaccine is first given? I think not. Aluminium allergy is known to be associated with an increased risk of developing atopic dermatitis or eczema (18), yet we are not told about it or tested for it. There are also other issues with aluminium that I will also discuss in Chapter 12 when we address toxicity.

The procession of moving through the stages from genetic susceptibility to hyperimmune reactivity and finally to allergic disease manifestations is modulated by environmental factors. (16) It is not just the environment around your cells (epigenetics), as we spoke about in Chapter 6, but also the potential allergens in your surrounding environment that can breach the skin barrier. Different people develop varying allergies primarily due to the potential allergens in their environment, which consequently breach the skin barrier.

Scientific findings continue to underline the importance of having an effective skin barrier to prevent allergic responses from developing due to antigens, allergens, and chemicals entering the skin and triggering the immune system. As we have already seen, Staphylococcus aureus acts as a persistent super-antigen activating the thymic stromal lymphopoietin cycle and stimulating IgE antibody production. It is also a known irritant, which is highly inflammatory when colonising atopic skin. (16)

So how do you prevent the Allergic March from developing? Quite simply, once these cycles are in play, the hyper-responsiveness of the immune system, the Th2 dominance, and high levels of IgE antibody production and inflammatory cytokines, it means that your body is primed to over-react with 'friendly fire' against any other similar proteins than infiltrate your damaged skin barrier. You may not be able to prevent it entirely once eczema has developed, but you can certainly slow it down and work to reduce the permeability of the skin and the number of antibodies in the system. As soon as a child develops excessively dry skin, all efforts should be taken to help support the skin barrier function to prevent the entry of potential allergens. If we do not take adequate measures to correct the skin barrier, increasing numbers of allergens and antigens penetrate it, resulting in the Allergic March. Coupled with Th2 polarisation, IgE antibody switching, and mast cell priming, eczema sufferers are perfectly ambushed for consequent allergic responses. However, we can fight back if we have the correct knowledge.

Once a person is caught in the eczema cycles, it is counterproductive to simply prescribe medications, steroids, and even immunological drugs if you have not first identified the irritants, such as allergic triggers. This allergic cycle is so prevalent in eczema that patients must be evaluated for allergies as quickly as possible. Appropriate action can then be taken to remove those allergens and reduce the resulting antibody production. (16) Otherwise, you will be fighting a losing and frustrating battle. Regarding allergy testing, if your finances permit and you want a complete picture, you can request skin prick tests, blood tests, and stool tests to cover all the different antibodies. However, do not negate the simple and cheap food tracker. Although allergy testing is good and can be necessary to identify potentially life-threatening allergens and sensitivities we may not have considered, our body is the most accurate measure of whether something agrees with us or not. Learning to listen to your body and to recognise patterns in your symptoms up to 72 hours after ingesting food will provide a much more accurate picture of sensitivities, which cause varying levels of inflammation but can have far-reaching and damaging consequences.

Therefore, the question is: can we do anything to arrest the Allergic March? Thankfully, the answer is yes.

Firstly, the previously mentioned histidine is not only responsible for carrying water up through the layers of the skin, but it also helps to regulate the histamine levels in your blood. Insufficient levels of histidine can result in abnormal histamine synthesis. We already know that histamine is the substance produced by the cells during allergic reactions and that eczema sufferers typically have higher histamine levels than people without eczema. Thus, you do not need any extra histamine as an eczema patient.

However, just as inflammation is a good thing when it works correctly, so is histamine. We do not need to eliminate it; we must maintain the correct levels. It is involved in many helpful reactions in the body. For example, histamine is essential to produce adequate hydrochloric acid in the stomach, to regulate the dilation of blood vessels and the microcirculation in muscles during exercise and is highly effective as both an antioxidant and anti-inflammatory agent. In addition, histamine helps to promote sleep and wakefulness by interacting with receptors in the brain.

The amino acid histidine helps to regulate more than just histamine and skin moisture. Therefore, insufficient histidine intake leads to more issues than only poor water binding in keratinocyte cells and histamine irregularities. Histidine deficiency has been shown to cause a deterioration in mood state and mental performance in humans, as well as causing anxiety-like symptoms in mice. Conversely, histidine supplementation has been shown to improve fatigue symptoms, filaggrin formation, cognitive and neurological performance, and numerous medical conditions such as atopic dermatitis (eczema), rheumatoid arthritis, inflammatory bowel disease, metabolic syndrome, and obesity. It has also been shown to suppress certain cancer cells and restore vision in mice with cataracts. (52) Furthermore, in all studies, histidine supplementation has been proven safe and effective without any adverse side effects, apart from in patients with liver disease. Hopefully, you do not need any more convincing to take histidine supplementation seriously. You can purchase histidine in 500g and 1 kg bags from bulk fitness and body-building supplements suppliers. If you do suffer from liver disease, you must seek advice from your medical practitioner regarding histidine supplementation. Still, I recommend you print the research documents and take them with you, as, unfortunately, a vast number of doctors have never even heard of histidine supplementation for eczema. If you bring this research to their attention and they start to recommend it, you could inadvertently help other eczema sufferers too.

There can be another issue going on inside people who display symptoms of histamine-mediated reactions, which is not directly due to type 1 allergies. To effectively regulate the amount of histamine in the blood, we need to produce an optimal amount of two particular enzymes: diamine oxidase (DOA) and N-methyl transferase. Diamine oxidase is considered to clear the excess histamine in our bodies that comes from certain foods we eat. N-methyl transferase helps to maintain the correct levels of histamine inside the cells and to mop it up after it is released following degranulation. (53, 61). However, if you develop a deficiency in the amino acids required to make these enzymes or a gene mutation that adversely affects your ability to produce these enzymes, your blood levels of histamine will rise higher than normal. This will lead to a condition called histamine intolerance. The human diamine oxidase gene is located on chromosome 7. Studies have found various mutations in this gene, which are associated with inflammatory diseases such as food allergy, gluten-sensitive enteropathy, Crohn's disease, ulcerative colitis, and colon adenoma, as well as some gastrointestinal diseases involving both benign and malignant tumour growths. Certain medications can also hinder diamine oxidase production. For example, metformin, commonly prescribed to lower blood sugar levels in type 2 diabetes, has been found to also target diamine oxidase receptors in the gut. (54) As diamine oxidase inhibits the ability of histamine to pass through the gut lining into the bloodstream, hindering either diamine oxidase production or diamine oxidase receptors will lead to raised histamine levels in the blood. (53) Therefore, a diamine oxidase deficiency could also be implicated in leaky gut syndromes in addition to histamine intolerance.

People suffering from histamine intolerance can typically display symptoms of allergic reactions, such as itching and eczema flares to some foods that naturally contain high levels of histamine. It is not a type 1 allergic reaction involving degranulation of cells, but rather that the levels of histamine in the body rise to levels that trigger allergy-like symptoms simply because of an inability to break down the excess histamine in those foods. According to the Healthline website, the following foods either contain high amounts of histamine or encourage the release of histamine in the body.

- Fermented foods, including cheese and alcohol (anaerobically fermented foods do not increase histamine, but care must be taken to ensure the food remains under the brine level, otherwise the presence of oxygen will cause histamine to develop)
- Dried fruits
- Avocados
- The nightshade family: tomatoes, eggplant, peppers, chilis, and in some cases, potatoes
- Spinach
- Processed or smoked meats
- Shellfish
- Bananas and plantain

- Wheatgerm
- Beans
- Papaya
- Chocolate
- Citrus fruits
- Nuts (particularly peanuts, cashews, and walnuts)

Alcohol, high-energy drinks, and green and black teas also block the production of the diamine oxidase enzyme in the gut, which is required to break down histamine.

As chronic eczema sufferers already have an excess of histamine due to the nature of the disease and the repeated degranulation of immune cells, they do not require additional histamine either from histamine-containing/promoting foods or from being unable to breakdown the histamine in their food. Does this mean that you need to avoid these foods? No, it does not. Forewarned is forearmed, as the saying goes. You must be aware of these foods and the possibility of you having a histamine intolerance reaction to assess your own symptoms and track how you respond to certain foods. As this type of reaction does not involve antibodies, it will not give a positive result on any allergy tests, but you will be able to see your reactions on a food tracker. I recommend you complete this tracker for at least one week. Record everything you eat or drink, along with the date and time. Each time you log an entry, record how your skin feels and how you feel emotionally on a scale of 1-5, with one being terrible and five being fantastic. If you can do this diligently for one week, you will see patterns occurring with rapid or delayed reactions to foods you have received negative allergy test results for. You will then know which foods are likely offenders. You should then remove them for a while to see if there is an improvement in your symptoms. Then you can re-introduce them to see if the suspected reaction is confirmed. However, please note that when re-introducing, you must only re-introduce one food at a time; otherwise, the results will be difficult to ascertain. Alternatively, a preferable option if you already display symptoms of other inflammation or autoimmune disease is to remove all of the most inflammatory foods for one month to heal the leaky gut and allow the antibodies in your circulation to reduce. Care must be taken with this approach, as removing too many foods at once can cause nutritional deficiencies, skewing your results and making it unclear which foods were causing you a problem. My personal preference is for you to eat your regular diet and grade your skin condition. An excellent resource to help with this protocol is a book by Amy Myers, M.D., titled The Autoimmune Solution Cookbook. This book provides nutritionally balanced meal plans and recipes, free from all potential autoimmune-triggering foods.

As food sensitives can cause many other inflammatory symptoms, you would also benefit from recording additional biomarkers too, such as brain clarity, energy levels, anxiety, sex drive, bloating, and increased mucus in your nose and throat.

By using the tracker method, I observed all my children having eczema flare after I ate nightshades and citrus when breastfeeding. A pattern emerged with them drinking my milk and reacting 24 hours after I consumed these foods. They were not even eating the food themselves. After they had been weaned, eating wheat was seen to cause loose stools, inability to sit still or focus, and eczema flares within 48 hours of eating it. One of my children had an unusual reaction in that she could eat wheat if she was inactive, but if she did any physical exertion for up to 4 hours either before or after eating wheat, she would react with hives and swelling around her eyes and face. This type of reaction is incredibly challenging to spot without keeping a detailed tracker; it is too obscure to see the pattern without a record of what has been eaten. If exercise-induced allergic reactions are something you feel you may be suffering from, you can read more about it in the articles I have referenced (62, 63, 64) but please also discuss this with your physician. Exercise can increase histamine levels in the blood by degranulating mast cells. If the levels are already elevated, possibly from recent exposure to environmental or food sensitivities, then it is possible that histamine toxicity or anaphylaxis-type reactions can occur. If you are already aware that certain foods can trigger this delayed reaction, then it would be prudent to either avoid those food triggers entirely or, at the very least, avoid any form of exercise from 6 hours before to 6 hours after consuming them.

Unless you are experiencing symptoms of autoimmune disease, which necessitates an ambitious approach to gain rapid results, keeping a tracker is a much less aggressive initial option. Strictly limiting yourself to only a few sparse non-allergenic foods and gradually introducing suspected offenders back one by one can be laborious and challenging. Furthermore, without expert nutritional guidance, following such a restrictive eating method can lead to nutritional deficiencies, which can also cause symptoms of their own, thus making your results difficult to interpret. Using the food tracker may take some effort, but you do not restrict any foods. On the contrary, you need to eat your regular diet for it to work.

Regarding food allergies, you should be aware that genetically modified or bioengineered foods are up to 11 times more allergenic than non-genetically modified foods. Furthermore, food additives can cause allergies too, particularly artificial colours and flavour enhancers. Most medical practitioners do not routinely test for these. Always check your labels: "If in doubt, throw it out" is a good motto. Clean food is better for the body, which is another reason to buy organic produce as much as possible or grow your own. I encourage you to read the following excellent blog article about food additives, published by Green Med Info in August 2018.

https://www.greenmedinfo.com/blog/ten-thousand-chemicals-food-and-food-packaging-what-are-these-substances-doing-our-children

I used the food tracker method to discover nearly all my children's allergies before they were even tested. It was what prompted one of the top allergy consultants in the world to be so impressed by my diagnostics that he asked me which branch of the medical profession I worked in before having my children. You can imagine his shock when I told him I had no medical background at all. It supports one of my favourite mantras: "Desperate mums do amazing things!" I was a desperate mum, and that desperation spurred me on to uncover what was happening inside my children and find ways to help them.

Anything that helps us restore balance naturally is a very welcome addition. If you have not already started taking an amino acid supplement to support your body, please consider doing so. Enzymes are made from amino acids, and by taking them, you can provide your body with the extra support it needs to produce vital enzymes for body functions, including diamine oxidase and N-methyl transferase. In addition, print the scientific documents and discuss with your doctor the merits of taking histidine to improve the water-carrying capabilities of your skin cells, along with its myriad of other health-enhancing benefits. Bear in mind that the longer food is present in the body, the more histamine it produces. Therefore, constipation will also increase histamine levels, so make every effort to eat enough fibre-containing foods, drink enough water, and exercise enough to keep your bowel movements regular. Your gut moves when you do.

Vitamin C is a natural antihistamine when taken at sufficient doses. Unfortunately, there is likely more incorrect and misleading information published about vitamin C than any other vitamin. I highly recommend reading '**Vitamin C: The Real Story**' by Steve Hickey, PhD, and Dr Andrew Saul, PhD, to discover accurate and science-based information. I experienced the antihistamine power of vitamin C shortly after reading that book. We were travelling in Trinidad, West Indies, and got stuck in terrible traffic on the highway. As we sat there, wondering how long it would take to start moving again, one of my children looked at her younger sibling and cried out, "Wow, look at your face! What did you eat?"

We turned round in our seats to see, and sure enough, my child was breaking out in hives around her mouth and eyes, which was typical of a nut reaction. She had not eaten anything out of the ordinary, and we still have no idea what caused the reaction. However, I was not unduly concerned at first. I routinely carry antihistamine medication in my handbag, so I was confident of being able to contain the reaction. Then I reached into my bag to take out the medicine and realised, to my dismay, it was not there. Someone had taken it out to rub onto a mosquito bite and had not put it back. I felt terrible for not having checked before we left home. My mind raced, trying to think of what to do. I had no idea where the nearest pharmacy was, and with us stuck in a seeming gridlock, I realised I would not be able to get to it anyway. Then I remembered reading Steve Hinkley and Andrew Saul's book, which proved vitamin C works as an excellent antihistamine if taken in high enough doses. I did have a bottle of chewable 500 mg vitamin C tablets in my bag. I took out eight tablets and handed them to my daughter, who was seven years old at the time, telling her to eat them all as quickly as possible. She did so willingly because she liked their orange flavour, and sure enough, within 5 minutes, every hive was gone. That shocked me. From then on, I kept my children on high-dose vitamin C (around 2000 mg daily in divided doses); they became much less reactive. Although I still carry the antihistamine medication, vitamin C is now my first response to any early allergy symptoms. However, such symptoms have been few and far between since we started the daily vitamin C regime.

Despite articles online stating that high doses of vitamin C are a waste of money because they pass out of the body in your urine, the opposite is true. Vitamin C is a highly effective natural treatment for many different ailments. If the argument about peeing out vitamin C were valid, then by the same reasoning, we may as well not drink water either because the more you drink, the more you pee out. We all know that drinking water is good for us and that it enters every part of our body to hydrate and cleanse before being passed out, and the same is true for vitamin C. As I am not writing a book about vitamin C, I will leave it that regular doses of vitamin C divided throughout the day should be a part of your antihistamine protocol. I gave my children high-dose vitamin C to reduce their eczema and allergic tendencies (around 2000 mg daily). I still give them around 5000 mg daily when they are unwell by making a drink from ascorbic acid powder mixed in water with sodium bicarbonate added at about 2:1 ratio (ascorbic acid: sodium bicarbonate) to reduce the acidity. I top it up with a little juice to make a pleasant, high-dose, fizzy vitamin C fruit drink. I follow the same ratio for myself but take higher doses of around 10,000 mg daily, increasing to 45,000 mg if I am fighting an illness. In Dr Saul's book, you can read more about the myriad health benefits associated with the often maligned but almost miraculous vitamin C. Alternatively, check out the science documents that are available at the Orthomolecular Society website (http://orthomolecular.org)

Thirdly, a natural herbal remedy, Mangifera indica, is used in Cuba to treat allergies, asthma, and eczema. It has been scientifically shown to reduce Th2 dominance, IgE levels, the allergic response of B and helper T cells, and the degranulation of mast cells, which results in a consequent lowering of histamine levels. (48, 49) Other studies have also found that Mangifera indica effectively reduces *Staphylococcus* infections due to its potent antibacterial properties. Furthermore, it promotes wound healing, particularly in skin conditions such as eczema and psoriasis. (50, 51) Trials have also shown increased cognitive performance equivalent to caffeine but without the negative effects. It achieves all this without pharmaceutical-like side effects! Why are patients not informed about these natural solutions?

Mangifera indica is made from the young leaves of the mango tree. You can purchase it in supplement form and tincture. It is freely available from herbalists and online, but in nations where mango trees grow, the young leaves can be picked and made into tea, cooked in soups and stews, added to salads and smoothies, or dried and powdered to take as a supplement. With such powerful medicinal benefits, this is one to consider adding to your routine.

After discussing the allergic cycle, you can see how the heightened immune response triggers the allergic tendency and re-enforces the suppression of S100 skin protein gene expression on the eczema spider web. In addition, the restricted dietary choices of those on the Allergic March easily cause nutritional deficiencies, further exacerbating dry skin. Elevated stress also has detrimental effects on your skin. Living with the constant fear of either exposure to allergic triggers or not being able to partake in certain activities or events due to the risk of exposure causes your stress levels to be higher than they should be and creates a cascade of undesirable responses. We will discuss the effects of stress in depth in a later chapter.

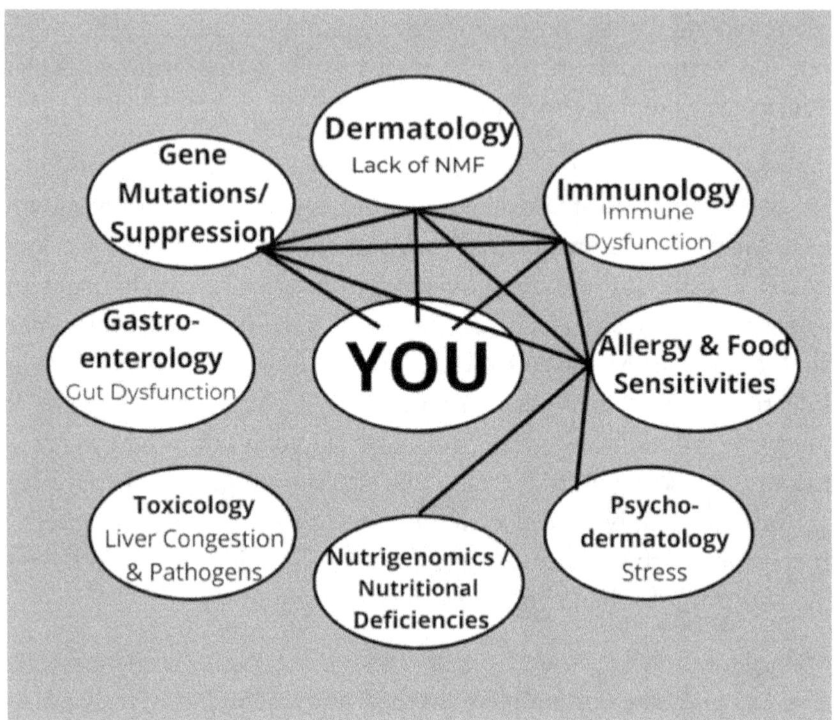

In the next chapter, I reveal which nutritional deficiencies are known to be involved in eczema development and severity.

Your action points for this chapter are listed on the next page.

Action points

1. Start completing the food tracker for at least three days, preferably one week.

2. Take supplemental vitamin C from non-genetically modified pure ascorbic acid powder. (Mix with sodium bicarbonate in a 2:1 ratio and flavour it with your favourite pure fruit juice.)

3. Consider taking Mangifera indica supplements or tea, or if you live in areas where mangos grow naturally, harvest some of the young leaves to use in salads and teas.

9

Feeding Healthy Skin

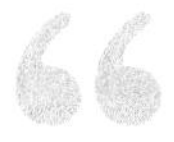

We dashed frantically from the cars and ran through the airport, sprinting to the check-in desk with cases half flying behind us, passports and tickets already in hand, hoping to claw back every valuable minute. We were finally here at the airport but groaned in desperation as we surveyed the queues at the check-in desks. Could we get this close and still miss our flight?

Back in 2018, after a 3-week sabbatical from the mission field, we arranged with a local pastor to help with transport for our return trip to Heathrow airport. One of the disciples would collect us at 5 am and drive the six of us in the church minibus with all our copious luggage. Right on time, the brother arrived at the hotel, and we duly loaded the suitcases, flight cases, and sleepy children into the back of the van. After ensuring all the kids' seatbelts were strapped, the minibus pulled away, only to splutter, jerk, and stall barely 20 feet down the road. To no avail, we checked everything we could think of and tried every possible solution to restart the minibus; however, we finally had to admit that the engine was flat-line DEAD! With flitting thoughts regarding the urgency of getting to the airport, our phone calls to arrange alternative transport became increasingly urgent. Everyone we called either had a vehicle too small to take us, or they already needed it to get to work and could not risk driving us themselves for fear of arriving back late. Time ticked incessantly away. We eventually managed to borrow the pastor's car and found a second vehicle and driver to take us all on the frantic dash to Heathrow. The minibus was pushed to the side of the road to await the tow truck.

On talking to our friend (who shall remain nameless) about the events leading up to his arrival at the hotel, he mentioned the minibus had been running fine, and he knew it was not due to lack of fuel as he had stopped on route to our hotel to fill the fuel tank with petrol. Before we left for missionary service, my husband had driven this particular minibus for many years, and he immediately picked up what our friend said.

"Hold on", he interjected. "Are you sure you put petrol in? It is a diesel engine!"

Sure enough, that is precisely what happened. The brother had filled the fuel tank with petrol instead of diesel, causing the engine to seize up completely. Surprisingly, the minibus had run fine from the service station to the hotel, but this was likely caused by the engine using the remnants of the previous fuel load. When the system encountered the wrong fuel, one it was not designed to utilise, the vehicle could no longer function and spluttered to a halt. And there lies the analogy with our bodies. When we fill up with the wrong type of fuel, we may be able to run for a little way with everything looking fine, but eventually, that unsuitable fuel works its way into our system, and we can no longer function as we should. Then things start to go awry, and some processes may even seize up completely.

Just so I do not leave you hanging, yes, we did make it to the airport in time, albeit having to run from security to the boarding lounge, dragging the four kids, six suitcases, and six flight cases along most comically. It reminded me of the airport scene from the original Home Alone movie.

Food is far more than just a means to remove hunger, just as fuel needs to do more than fill up a tank. Over the years, I have heard many people state: "You are what you eat." However, I disagree. It is far more accurate to say: "You are what you absorb." It is the nutrients we ABSORB that feed our cells and our body, not just the food that passes through our digestive tract. This leads us to consider not just the nutritional content of the food we eat but also whether we can utilise those nutrients effectively. Just as you cannot expect the diesel engine in your vehicle to run efficiently on petrol, similarly, you cannot expect your body to function at optimal health if you fuel yourself with foods devoid of nutrients. It simply will not have the elements necessary to thrive.

What type of fuel or food are we humans designed to eat? Well, our teeth resemble other primates in the animal kingdom, and we also share many similarities in our DNA. Some vegan advocates use this similarity to claim we should eat a herbivore diet like primates. But if we look at the chimpanzee's diet as an example of a primate diet, we will see that they are not actually vegans.

Yes, when fruit is in short supply, chimpanzees will also eat flowers and tree bark and having sweet loving taste buds like many of us, they are also rather partial to honey. Contrary to popular belief, though, chimpanzees do not just eat bananas and fruit. They also supplement their diet with lizards, eggs, and insects, such as ants and termites, and occasionally hunt for small animals to eat. Their diet typically consists of only around 6% derived from animal sources, which makes them omnivores, not herbivores.

My bookshelf is filled with health books from various disciplines, but a few stand out as my favourites. They are exceptional works backed by much scientific research and are very educational. One, '**The China Study**' by T. Colin Campbell, PhD and Thomas M. Campbell II, MD, exposes the health effects of diets worldwide. It highlights the stark differences in health and disease between those who adhere to more indigenous diets and those who adopt the typical standard American or Westernized diet. The areas around the world with the best health and the highest numbers of centenarians (people who live past 100 years old) are called blue zones. One common trait observed in these blue zones is that the amount of animal products consumed is typically less than 10% of the dietary intake. Instead, their diet is very much plant-based but not entirely vegan. The most common denominators in the blue zone diets are eating lots of beans, greens, tubers (root vegetables), nuts, and whole grains (such as oats). In addition, other similarities exist between those living in the blue zones that do not relate to diet but more to the social and environmental aspects of life, such as living in supportive communities and families. They also tend to live in areas with plenty of sunshine, and they spend a good proportion of their time outside interacting with nature, often the ocean, forests, or their gardens, while growing their own crops. While this chapter is primarily about nutrition, bear in mind that these other aspects of life also need to be considered. We will talk about these more in Chapter 11.

Regarding diet, eczema sufferers need to take particular care to ensure they are feeding healthy skin, particularly from the point of view of obtaining adequate amino acids and avoiding foods that can cause further inflammation. Our diet predominantly creates the ideal environment for the correct gut microbiome to flourish, impacting our immune system's efficiency and ability to detoxify. Those consuming more ancestral diets in the blue zones do not tend to deal with depleted microbiomes, toxic overload, excess inflammation, or allergic tendencies. For this reason, their bodies can tolerate things like lectins in nuts, seeds, and legumes, which can be problematic for those who have already developed chronic inflammatory and auto-immune diseases. Lectins not only cause gut irritation in susceptible individuals, but they are also commonly called anti-nutrients as they bind to minerals and prevent their absorption, increasing the risk of nutritional deficiencies. Blue zone areas do not typically use legumes in the form of mass-produced, tinned beans but of the dried variety, which are properly prepared. Canned beans are often blanched and then packed into their cans with water, salt, and often other chemicals to help them maintain their colour and texture. They are then steamed at high temperatures.

In contrast, in areas where people follow indigenous diets, dried beans are soaked overnight at a minimum and often for 24-48 hours before cooking. The skins are sometimes rubbed off and discarded. The beans are boiled at a high temperature for around 15 minutes before simmering until they are soft, which will vary depending on the bean but typically takes many hours. The alternative and preferred cooking method is to use a pressure cooker, which is the most effective way to reduce lectins and other anti-nutrients. You can also blend the soaked beans into a paste with seasonings and make some form of steamed or fried dumpling-type recipe. The indigenous method of soaking, sometimes skinning and boiling, reduces the anti-nutrients mostly present in the skins of beans and legumes. Pressure cooking or slow cooking reduces the remnant even further. You can also reduce lectins and anti-nutrients by sprouting the beans after the soaking process or by Lacto-fermenting them. These blue zone areas eat lots of beans but consume much fewer lectins from them. Our preference for convenience comes at a price! Not everyone has a noticeable problem with beans or lectins. Still, you should be aware of the possibility of them increasing inflammation, especially if your gut is already inflamed and leaking, which in cases of eczema is highly likely! Keep the food tracker record and if you do eat beans, nuts, or seeds, make sure you prepare them properly. Dried beans should be soaked for 1-2 days, changing the water frequently (removing the skins is optional), then rapidly boiling for 10-15 minutes before simmering until the beans are soft or adding to the pressure cooker. You can lower the lectin content in nuts and seeds by soaking them overnight and removing the skins or outer husks containing most of the lectin. Tinned produce should really be avoided as it is not appropriately prepared to remove anti-nutrients. They also risk chemical contamination from the tins and liners, especially if the cans are damaged. Convenient is not usually healthy, unfortunately!

In his excellent book '**Regenerate**', Sayer Ji confirms similar findings: indigenous diets provide the nutrients to promote health and wellness, and standard Westernized diets promote disease and sickness. He writes that we must consider what our ancestors ate, not try to copy what works for everyone else. He teaches that we have our own genetic code derived from our personal ancestors, and it is that code which determines the most health-promoting diet for us, not a video on social media of someone promoting what worked for them. For example, if your ancestors grew up in a Caribbean village eating home-reared chickens, green leaves, and root vegetables, that will likely be your most healthful diet. In contrast, someone of Eskimo descent will more likely thrive on a diet high in cold water or oily fish.

In both the books mentioned above, some common threads also bear out in my own experience. One of those is that we do need to focus on eating more fresh local plants and discipline ourselves to eat less processed junk food. I am repeatedly drumming into my children one dietary mantra: "Something raw with every meal!" Why do I say this? Because raw foods are high in vitamins and minerals that nourish our bodies. They also contain other compounds called antioxidants, enzymes, phytochemicals, and microRNAs, which are essential for our health. We neglect these dietary pearls at our peril. Let us look at what these substances are and why you need them.

Antioxidants

Oxidation is constantly occurring within our bodies as a byproduct of living; however, it increases when we are exposed to toxins or stress. Oxidation is the name given to when molecules lose electrons to another substance, termed the oxidising agent (the one that takes the electrons away). Losing these electrons causes molecules to become unstable. You can see oxidation in action when you cut an apple and leave it open to the air. As it loses electrons, it starts to turn brown. Vitamin C is an effective antioxidant. It prevents oxidation, which you can see work when you rub a cut apple or avocado with freshly squeezed lemon juice; they will not turn brown. The antioxidant power of vitamin C in the lemon protects them from oxidation. With apples, we may not worry about it too much, but when the molecules in our body oxidise and lose electrons, it makes them less able to function optimally. DNA and proteins are molecules too, and it stands to reason that we need these to perform well for us to be in good health.

You may have heard of free radicals. They are typically given bad press and accused of damaging our bodies and being the source of all oxidation events. They indeed do cause oxidation, but if kept in the correct proportions, free radicals are helpful to the body for proper function. They play essential roles in regulating cell signalling in multiple areas. When we live a healthy lifestyle and eat a diet with sufficient antioxidants, our body can scavenge the free radicals and keep oxidation levels within the correct range. However, when the levels of free radicals in the body rise to excess, it becomes too much for the body to deal with, and then oxidative stress occurs. This is when free radicals start becoming detrimental to our health. Many scientific studies have linked oxidative stress with the development and progression of many diseases, such as, but not limited to, cancer, heart disease, diabetes, metabolic diseases, and accelerated ageing. This is due to the unstable molecules being unable to function as they should, so processes and functions in the body start to break down.

You may be wondering where these free radicals come from. Well, we produce some of them ourselves when we have inflammation, infection, stress, or even by exercising excessively. Unless these are chronic long-term events, our body will be able to cope with these and use its reactive oxygen species scavenging systems to keep things under control. Unfortunately, though, free radical production also occurs when we are exposed to environmental pollutants such as medications, heavy metals, processed and fried foods, chemical exposures, pesticides, cigarette smoke, air pollution, alcohol, radiation, and electromagnetic fields (EMF), to name a few. (57) When you consider the amount of environmental pollution we currently live with and the Western diet we consume, it is far more than our innate ability to keep in check. This means we lose electrons faster than we can replace them, and unstable molecules start wreaking havoc inside us. I have devoted a whole chapter to toxic overload. For now, just understand that our bodies need help to deal with the onslaught of pollution we live with.

Time for the antioxidant superheroes to enter the show. Raw plants contain antioxidants. Plants cannot pick themselves up and move home when they do not like their surroundings. They will either die if their circumstances have become too dire, or they will produce antioxidants, phytochemicals, and microRNAs to adapt and survive. These compounds then become beneficial to us in mopping up the free radicals, repairing the damage, and communicating with our cells on how to adapt to our own environment. Antioxidants are called such because they carry 'spare' electrons and donate them back to our molecules, restabilising them again. Thus, antioxidants help to repair oxidation, hence their name, which means 'against oxidation'.

Phytochemicals are another compound produced by plants as they adapt to protect themselves against damage by bacteria, fungi, and attacks by insects. The phytochemicals give plants their distinct colours; plants' antioxidant and phytochemical composition varies depending on their colour. Consequently, differently coloured plants contain a vast array of healing compounds, which is why we are encouraged to eat a wide variety of coloured plants in our diets. This provides us with an abundance of health-promoting and healing compounds. For example, plant phenolic compounds from tea and berries are reported to have antimicrobial properties, which help to modulate the gut microbiota in humans, contributing to maintaining the correct balance between pathogenic and commensurate or friendly organisms. The anthocyanins from berries have also been shown to be effective in suppressing the growth of pathogenic *Staphylococcus, Salmonella, Bacillus cereus,* and *Helicobacter pylori* in the gut. (44)

Eating chlorophyll from green plants causes our bodies to interact with sunlight exposure differently, producing many health benefits. Chlorophyll protects the body from damage caused by ultraviolet light. Therefore, chlorophyll and sunlight work in harmony. Consuming green plants without exposing the body to natural sunlight will not reap the full benefits of chlorophyll in producing energised water or coenzyme Q10, even though the antioxidant and nutritional benefits will still be the same. Similarly, sunlight exposure without the consumption of chlorophyll leaves a lack of protection against the damaging effects of ultraviolet light. The threat of skin damage may be caused not so much by excess sun exposure but by exposure in the absence of protective chlorophyll from eating green plants.

To maximise your consumption of antioxidants and phytochemicals, eat rainbows. Young children are happy to join in the rainbow eating challenge. Put a chart on the wall or fridge and challenge them to eat two different fruits or vegetables in each of five different colours to achieve a reward each day. You will significantly help the nutritional profile of your children. As adults, though, we must not neglect ourselves or forget that we need rainbows as much as children do, possibly more as we deal with the effects of ageing.

Probiotics and Prebiotics

Fresh raw foods contain anti-inflammatory probiotics too. Picking berries straight from the garden, salads, or herbs you grew on the windowsill, and especially raw foods that have been Lacto-fermented, provides your gut with much-needed friendly microbes to repopulate the gut microflora. As we saw in Chapter 9, our microbiome is under constant assault from our modern lifestyle, so eating probiotic-containing foods is essential to avoid microbes becoming depleted.

Fermenting foods multiplies the probiotics in them. Whereas probiotic supplements can contain between one and 24 different strains of bacteria, in contrast, there are around 2,000 different strains of probiotic organisms in half a cup of kimchi. Fermenting food yourself is also much more cost-effective than purchasing expensive probiotic supplements every month. Those with eczema need to ensure they ferment foods only in anaerobic environments. This means that they must be in air-tight containers (with the gas released by loosening the top a few times a day to avoid the containers bursting open), with the food kept submerged under the brine, usually by pressing it down with fermenting weights. Ferments in contact with the air contain increased amounts of histamine, which can cause symptoms of histamine release, such as those occurring in histamine intolerance for those who already have raised histamine levels. Anaerobic ferments do not have high histamine levels and are much safer for eczema sufferers if they are prepared and stored correctly.

When consuming probiotic foods or supplements, it is also essential to create the ideal environment in the gut for them to flourish. If they arrive in a barren landscape and are given nothing to help them survive, they will die, and all your efforts will be in vain.

Probiotics need prebiotics to consume. Prebiotics are indigestible starches and fibres in root vegetables and complex carbohydrate foods. They provide the necessary fermentable products the probiotics need to thrive. Through fermentation, they release compounds that heal us as they digest them.

The gut bacteria also digest and break down almost all kinds of amino acids. The fermentation bi-products of the microbes digesting these amino acids and indigestible starches from plant foods include short-chain fatty acids and branched-chain fatty acids. These are essential for maintaining a healthy gut lining and producing adequate neurotransmitters to maintain optimal brain and emotional function. (44) People who suffer from anxiety and depression often have a problem with their gut, not a problem with their brain. Lacking the microbes that produce short-chain fatty acids, such as serotonin, means that the brain is deprived of the materials it needs to regulate our emotions and to feel calm.

We have already spoken of probiotics and their importance in regulating the inflammatory response of your immune system. Creating the right environment for your friendly gut microbes to flourish is vital, especially when dealing with a chronic inflammatory condition such as eczema. Eating correctly is your primary way to achieve this.

MicroRNA

Another vital substance in raw plants is microRNA. RNA is the copy of various parts of the DNA code. In Chapter 6, I spoke of DNA being like the main instruction manual and RNA as the copies made to carry out specific instructions. Plants have DNA just like we do; therefore, they also have RNA, which means, by default, they also have microRNA. The microRNA is produced in the plants to help them adapt to their environment. It binds to the coding portion of the RNA and influences how the instruction is carried out.

When we eat raw plants, their microRNAs act like messengers to our cells. They survive our digestive processes and, once absorbed, can travel to our cells and convey necessary instructions regarding how we need to adapt to our environment. They do this by binding to the coding portion of the RNA that is produced when we copy the instructions from our DNA. They then regulate how our genes function (whether they are turned on or off/up or down). According to an article published on MDPI.com, microRNAs regulate at least 60%

of all gene expressions. (58) This is incredible! Something as simple as eating locally produced, fresh raw plants can influence how your genes are expressed, which directly impacts your disease susceptibility. Ginger, for example, has been shown to contain microRNAs that stimulate the growth of *Lactobacillus* microbes in the gut and help to reduce inflammation. (24) Ginger is well renowned and accepted as a natural anti-inflammatory food. It has been shown in scientific studies to inhibit the production of prostaglandins, leukotrienes, and TNF-α, which are all biomolecules that promote inflammation. (23)

MicroRNAs can enter our DNA code and influence how those codes express in much the same way as turning a key can open or close a lock. Therefore, eating locally-grown organic produce as much as possible is extremely important. These plants adapt within your local environment, so their messages are particularly pertinent to local people. When we do not eat plants (or we cook every vesture of life out of them), we deprive our body of these vital keys, the microRNAs and the information needed for our bodies to adapt effectively.

Another important issue concerning microRNA concerns the consequences we are reaping from tampering with the DNA in the plants we eat. This process is known as genetic engineering, or by its newer terms, bioengineering or transgenic. Genetic engineering was promoted as a solution to losing crops to common plant diseases and pests. By changing the DNA in the plant cells, usually by combining it with the DNA from a plant that is not susceptible to that disease or pest, agricultural scientists can create a hybrid version of the original plant, which is disease resistant, but still looks like the original. Plants are also genetically modified to allow them to survive the spraying of weedkillers, such as Roundup™ and Glyphosate. In theory, and if you accept it without considering further ramifications, it sounds like a helpful tool to increase farming efficiency. However, just as we are consistently learning that the human body is intertwined and cannot be separated into independent categories, so it is with the rest of the world too. You cannot tamper with something in one area of the body without releasing ramifications elsewhere. Similarly, we cannot tamper with the genetic makeup of plants and expect it to have no ramifications elsewhere in the food chain or environment. So what happens when we eat plants with altered DNA?

Well, I just spoke of the importance of the microRNA messenger system. RNA is copied from DNA; therefore, it is common sense that if you tamper with the DNA, the RNA copied from it will also be different. The plant may look the same to the naked eye, it may have the same nutritional profile of calories, carbohydrates, vitamins, and minerals, but if the RNA is altered, the unnatural microRNA will no longer fit the locks in our DNA to effectively control our gene expression. If the RNA is changed, the messages in the microRNA will also be altered, consequently starving our cells of the communication and nutrients they need to function. The antioxidant and phytochemical structure could also be changed as a result. As far as I am aware, no studies exist to show the long-term effects of consuming altered microRNAs and phytochemicals.

In his book '**Regenerate**', Sayer Ji likens microRNAs to software and the genetic code to hardware. The analogy is a good one. Depending on the software plugged into your computer, the functionality of your hardware is radically changed. Similarly, depending on the software of the microRNAs we plug into our bodies, the functionality of our DNA and gene expression will vary, either to promote our health and regeneration or to trigger our disease and demise. Such a choice is largely under our own control. We tamper with our food chain at our peril. The vast number of foods sold in stores that either contain or are contaminated by genetically modified ingredients is quite scary. It is equally frightening to see the increasing data showing an almost perfect correlation between escalating genetically modified foods and glyphosate spraying with escalating chronic diseases of all types. The only way to protect yourself is to grow your own or buy organically grown, at the very least, certified, non-genetically modified foods.

Similarly, many animals farmed for meat are genetically wired to require a plant-based diet and live in the sunshine, grazing, for optimal health. The sun on the plants creates chlorophyll, and the animals eat the plants and digest them, absorbing all the nutrients and microRNAs from them. When we eat the meat from these animals, we reap the benefits of the sunshine, chlorophyll, and nutrients in the animal. With the advent of industrialised intensive farming practices, animals have been moved out of their natural environment into cramped stalls, never grazing nor seeing the light of day, and being fed genetically engineered cereals, which are totally unnatural for the animal to eat. As a result, the animals are prone to disease and can be kept on antibiotics to mitigate the frequent infections. The resulting chronic inflammation and stress in the animals leads to the release of stress hormones, which promotes further inflammation and the accumulation of unhealthy fatty deposits as their bodies try to isolate the toxins. That is, without mentioning any hormones that may be fed to the animals to increase their weight and the subsequent price at market. Then we eat the meat from these animals (usually to excess) along with all their toxic overload and inflammation. Do you see why I recommend that any meat you eat be from pasture-reared, organically-raised animals?

Enzymes

Like us, raw plants also produce enzymes. We use them for a myriad of bodily functions, including, but not limited to, the manufacture of healthy skin, dealing with inflammation, and digesting food. Unfortunately, we can become less efficient at producing enzymes as we age. However, if we were to eat a healthy, predominantly plant-based diet, we would consume beneficial enzymes from the raw plants. These enzymes not only help us to break down the food we eat but also serve as functional elements in our diets to help facilitate many processes in the body. However, cooking and preservation destroy plant enzymes, so we must consciously consume a decent proportion of our plant foods in their raw state. Therefore, I tell my children to eat something raw with every meal.

Is a Vegan Diet Good for Healing Eczema?

Now that you know the importance of eating a wide variety of raw and cooked plants to obtain your antioxidants and phytochemicals and the dangers of eating industrialised animal products, do I recommend becoming strictly vegan? No, I do not, and this is not something I say lightly. There are many benefits to eating a predominantly plant-based diet and many ethical concerns over the treatment of animals, especially in industrialised farming. However, we are dealing with a particular health concern that requires adequate amounts of histidine and iron, along with many other nutrients necessary for skin health. The most readily absorbable forms of these nutrients are in meat. Vegans typically have far lower carnosine concentrations in their muscles than meat eaters. Histidine is released from carnosine, and to repeat what I stated earlier, histidine deficiency hinders the production of profilaggrin, filaggrin, and the natural moisturising factor, and has been shown to result in the development of eczema, even in those who do not have a genetic predisposition. (4)

In addition, strict vegans will also need to supplement with vitamin B12, docosahexaenoic acid (DHA) and eicosapentaenoic acid (EPA) from Omega 3 fats, which they would have obtained from eating oily fish. Furthermore, oily fish contains valuable amounts of vitamin D, especially for those who live in colder climates with limited ultraviolet exposure and who would struggle to manufacture enough vitamin D in the skin. However, as I just said, eating farmed animals and fish pumped full of synthetic estrogen, antibiotics, and an unnatural diet is not the best option for healthy eating. So, if you do eat meat, it should be as close to nature as possible: grass-fed, pasture-raised, and organically reared. Fish should be sourced from water with minimal pollution, preferably wild-caught Alaskan salmon, Pacific sardines, and farmed rainbow trout. Farmed Atlantic salmon is highly inflammatory due to the unnatural diet and environment of the fish and the colours fed to them to create what should have been the characteristic natural pink colour. In contrast, farmed rainbow trout are healthier than their wild relatives due to the pollution in the rivers where wild trout swim.

Many vegan plant-based products are not the health foods they are touted to be, being highly processed and often genetically modified meat and cheese substitutes. As such, they are highly inflammatory in the body. Junk food is still junk food, even when it is plant-based. Eat food as close to nature as possible, and you afford yourself much better protection for your diet and health.

Thus, we have established that eczema sufferers do need to eat meat. However, meat is devoid of fibre and passes through the intestinal tract much slower than plant foods. It also encourages the growth of pathogenic bacteria as it decays inside us. These microbes, in turn, produce ammonia compounds, which increase inflammation in the gut lining. Studies have shown there is a direct correlation between the amount of red meat a person consumes and their risk of developing colon cancer. (83) However, this is likely due to eating too little fibre and plant foods with meat to speed its transition through the gut and provide adequate antioxidants. Eating less red meat may be better for your health, depending on your genetic makeup, but removing meat altogether can bring more problems to the table when trying to heal eczema. Some people have healed their skin by eating an almost exclusively meat diet, which directly contradicts that "too much is bad for you" narrative. This leads to the question: how can we eat meat more healthily?

We should eat organic, grass-fed meat, clean, unpolluted fish, and lots of plants to provide antioxidants to mop up any free radicals and fibre to speed the transition through the gut. I also thoroughly clean the meat we eat according to old Biblical traditions. This involves soaking the meat in cold salt water for 30 minutes and then rinsing it three times in clean water. This reduces the bacterial load in the meat and makes it less inflammatory to eat. We also trim the excess fat off the meat (toxins tend to be stored in the fat) and supplement the meals with adequately prepared beans and plenty of vegetables to speed up the transition time through the digestive tract. This reduces the time available for pathogenic bacteria and ammonia compounds to be produced in the colon. Chunky root vegetable stews are an excellent way to combine meat with plenty of vegetables and beans. I like to use turkey or occasionally lamb, as they are both flavorful, and a little meat goes a long way in flavouring the whole meal. Although we do not tend to eat them raw, root vegetables contain wonderfully healthy fibres, starches, and complex carbohydrates that feed our microbiome. When we cook them in casseroles and soups, the cooking water is an integral part of the meal, and many of the phytochemical properties remain in the dish, rather than if you had boiled them and thrown away the cooking water. In addition, boiling meat in this way has been shown to produce fewer inflammatory compounds than if it is fried or roasted.

If you suffer from eczema, I do encourage you to consider your meat consumption. If you eat a lot of meat, you should be careful to consume sufficient plants to obtain fibre, antioxidants, phytochemicals and microRNA. If you are eating very little meat, your diet may contribute to deficiencies in the nutrients you receive from meat. I do not advise people to remove meat from their diet due to their necessity for extra histidine. White meats and clean fish have not been associated with increased cancer risk, so switching to more of these and consuming less red meat is an option if you are concerned about possible colon cancer. However, carnosine, from which histidine is derived, is far more abundant in red meat, so I would not advise removing red meat altogether.

Other nutrient deficiencies are also known to be implicated in the development of eczema. Many of these are also more readily available in meat, especially organ meats, as you will see later in this chapter. Instead, I encourage those I work with to eat at least ten portions of different coloured plant foods daily, emphasising eating plenty of green leaves to speed the transit time of waste through the gut. Beans and other pulses also increase the protein content of meals, but you must be careful to identify any sensitivity to lectins first or potential molecular mimicry. You may have to add beans to your diet slowly, assessing for gastrointestinal distress. In addition, soaking dried beans for 24-48 hours and then boiling rapidly for 10-15 minutes before simmering will reduce the compounds that cause the gassiness and break down the lectins, which act as anti-nutrients. If you still suffer from distention, gas, or other inflammatory gastrointestinal conditions or notice increased inflammation, you should remove lectin foods and focus on healing your gut.

Furthermore, it is wise to consider requesting IgG and IgA antibody testing for food sensitivities from your health professional.

Eating at least ten plant foods daily is easier than it sounds. For example, you can easily make a salad and a smoothie with five different plants in each. By doing this, you have achieved your ten already, without even counting the fruits or nuts (if you are not allergic to them) that you eat as snacks or vegetables with your evening meal.

For breakfast, I usually eat either a vegetable and fruit smoothie with added flax seeds or a bowl of porridge made with organic oats. When I eat porridge, I sweeten it by adding chopped organic dried fruits while cooking rather than adding sugar. Then once cooked and cooled a little, I add some almond butter or coconut cream to make it creamy as I do not eat dairy, plus a tablespoon of flax seeds and either hemp seeds or chia seeds, and then some cocoa to make it chocolate flavoured. (I have never really liked porridge, but once I realised it was good for me, I had to find a way to eat it. I love dark chocolate, so I figured I could enjoy it by making my porridge cocoa-heavy!) This breakfast provides me with five plant foods right at the start of the day, albeit not all raw. Flax seeds are a miracle plant that can help heal the gut. They are one of the best natural treatments for constipation as long as you drink sufficient water when consuming them. Organic oats also help heal the gut lining and contain valuable beta-glucans, which aid in maintaining a healthy heart. I only eat organic oats as tests on oat supplies showed that all oats were contaminated with glyphosate pesticide residues, apart from the organic brands.

Yes, eating in the manner I describe will take more preparation time. It will cost more, especially if you start buying organic, non-genetically modified plant foods and meat sourced from organic, pasture-raised animals, but is it worth it to help restore your health? Yes, it is. Your life is precious. You are worth every penny (or cent, depending on where you live). Personally, I would rather eat smaller portions of clean, high-nutrient-density foods that will nourish and heal me than fill up with high-toxicity, low-nutrient options that will starve my cells and increase inflammation in my body. Let us move on and look at supplements.

Nutritional Supplements

Although Orthomolecular Medicine and treating disease with mega doses of vitamins have been ridiculed in the past (primarily because it is a threat to certain industries' profits), evidence now shows that some people genuinely do need far higher nutrient levels than the standard recommended doses. This can be due to loss of function or null mutations in our gene expressions, malabsorption issues resulting from damaged brush borders in our gut lining, or gut dysbiosis resulting in a lack of bacterial pathways to synthesise the nutrients. Inadequate nutrient intake due to allergen avoidance can also lead to nutritional deficiencies. I reiterate we are what we absorb, not what we eat! For this reason, dietary supplements can provide vital support for the body to heal and function optimally.

Whilst I do believe that nutritional support should be an integral part of eczema healing, care should be taken to consult a qualified practitioner before self-medicating with high-dose supplements, especially if using other medications. Taking mega doses should be done with care, as some vitamins are fat soluble and are therefore stored by the body, which can lead to toxic levels building up. However, hundreds of research documents prove the efficacy and safety of many supplements when used at higher-than-normal doses. Comparing the safety records of mega-dose vitamin therapy to the safety records of pharmaceutical drugs makes it starkly evident which one is safer. It is also important to realise that the daily recommended doses for vitamin intake were the minimal doses necessary for sailors to avoid developing scurvy while at sea for long periods. They are not the doses recommended to help people achieve optimal health, and they take no account of the fact that when it comes to nutrition, there is no such thing as 'one size fits all'.

Eczema patients are often deficient in many nutrients when compared to 'normal' control subjects. It is highly probable that due to issues with their gut microbiome, eczema patients absorb fewer nutrients than they should. However, it is also equally possible that genetic mutations and higher levels of inflammation mean they require far more elevated amounts of these nutrients to function within the normal parameters. Studies have not been able to ascertain whether these deficiencies could contribute to the original development of eczema or whether they occur after a person develops eczema. It is like the "Which came first, the chicken or the egg?" scenario. Regardless of which way it is, these are the primary deficiencies you need to check for.

Iron

Iron-deficient anaemia is positively correlated with eczema. The inability to absorb iron efficiently has been implicated in developing many skin conditions, including eczema. (75) Iron deficiency adversely affects the ability of neutrophils and macrophages (innate immune cells) to effectively conduct their anti-bacterial activity, which then leads to increased colonisation of pathogenic bacteria such as the dreaded *Staphylococcus*. Iron is also necessary for the correct formation of skin, mucous membranes, hair, nails, and the tongue; changes in any of these should prompt medics to check for iron deficiency, especially as it is the most common deficiency in the world. (76) Symptoms of iron deficiency can include extreme fatigue, shortness of breath (due to reduced ability to transport oxygen), slow wound healing, brittle or spoon-shaped nails, reduced ability to fight infections and a pale complexion.

In food, iron is more readily available to the body in heme form, which comes from meat. Although some plants are also sources of iron, some people do not efficiently convert iron from the plant form and can become iron deficient on vegan diets. Regardless of ethical choices and ideals, we must never forget that people are individuals with unique genomes and microbiomes. For this reason, no one should ever assert that one diet is suitable for everyone. Remember, you are what you absorb, and your body's requirements may be different to the needs of others. Although many studies do recommend reducing your intake of animal products to less than 10% of your total food consumption due to the association of excess meat consumption with the development of many diseases, you do need to be aware that maintaining optimal iron levels is extremely important, especially if you have eczema. You can also increase the amount of iron you absorb by eating vitamin C sources while consuming iron.

If you establish that you are iron deficient, you should seek advice on supplementation to correct any deficiency. Iron is toxic when taken to excess, so you should seek medical guidance on the correct dosage. I prefer to work with nutritionists who can recommend iron supplements that do not irritate the gut or cause constipation. However, just because you are within the 'normal' range does not mean that you are not deficient. I know that sounds illogical. Let me share a personal experience to explain why I say this. I had a particularly rough labour with one of my babies, including shoulder dystocia, which required some almost violent interventions to get my daughter out before she was harmed from oxygen deprivation. In the process, I lost a large amount of blood, and the hospital considered giving me a transfusion. However, when they checked my blood, my iron levels were still within the normal range (10.8 g/dl), and consequently, I was told I did not need a transfusion after all. For the next few months, I was constantly sick. I seemed to have no immune strength and was repeatedly prescribed antibiotics for reoccurring *Staphylococcus* infections in my skin. Eventually, I saw a doctor who used her instinct instead of the computerised guidelines; she decided to check back through my medical history to see what my iron levels had been over my previous tests rather than comparing me to the 'normal' ranges. She was surprised to find that my normal haemoglobin levels were historically at the high end of normal (14.8 g/dl). This means I had lost almost 30% of my haemoglobin in one fell swoop, and consequently, my immune system was suffering. There I was, thinking my extreme fatigue was just the result of trying to cope with a newborn and a 1-year-old when I was actually suffering from anaemia symptoms. Even though my blood tests put me within the normal range, it was not normal for me and was causing me serious health issues. I am incredibly grateful my doctor used her common sense instead of sticking to the guidelines on her computer. You should always keep copies of your past test results and make sure you know your own numbers. You may spot something amiss when your doctor overlooks it because they focus only on checking whether you are within the given parameters and not whether your numbers have changed significantly for you.

Iron supplements can cause gastrointestinal distress, such as constipation. If you are advised to supplement, check for a product that is gentle on the gut. One of my favourite brands is Floravital. It is plant-based, does not cause constipation, and is also gluten-free.

Vitamin D3

Vitamin D is necessary for the correct formation of keratinocyte stem cells, as well as for immune function. Therefore, people with eczema should have blood tests to check their serum levels at the earliest opportunity, as vitamin D deficiency hinders the production of new skin cells at the earliest stages.

Vitamin D is also essential to maintain immune health. Those deficient in Vitamin D have a much higher risk of developing respiratory distress from illnesses such as seasonal flu or coronavirus. Skin infections can be more severe in those who are vitamin D deficient too. One of my children contracted a wart infection in the eczema on her hand, and her immune system was unable to deal with it because, unknown to me, she was vitamin D deficient. In a short time, she had over 40 warts on her hands and wrists. Our doctor expressed concern that she may have some type of immune disorder and said she needed to be referred to a specialist pediatric immunologist. However, before she was referred, I read an article on vitamin D deficiency and realised my mixed-race children were likely deficient, living with limited sun exposure in the United Kingdom. I promptly purchased a fish oil supplement for them. What happened next will shock you. All 40 warts disappeared after only two days of the fish oil supplementation! Yes, I said two days! There is no medication on earth that could have produced such amazing results in that time frame with no adverse side effects.

Other symptoms of vitamin D deficiency include deep bone pain, fatigue, muscle weakness, and depression. The goal of supplementation should be to raise your levels of D3 to the therapeutic or optimal range, not just an acceptable level. The best way to get vitamin D is to get into the sunlight. The sun converts cholesterol into vitamin D in the skin. However, not everyone gets to live in sunny climates, and eczema is generally more prevalent in countries with less sunshine. In these colder climates, the waters have more oily fish, which would provide adequate vitamin D if we ate an indigenous diet. Vitamin D supplementation will likely be necessary for those who cannot or do not wish to eat fish. When taking vitamin D supplements, look for D3 in the form of cholecalciferol, which is more readily absorbed by the body. Work with a professional who can regularly check your serum levels, as vitamin D is a fat-soluble vitamin that is stored in the body. Correcting a severe deficiency can take many months, but without checking, you could exceed what is optimal and pass into toxic levels. Any inflammation in the gut can also make it more difficult for you to absorb and use the vitamin D in supplement form, and you may need to take much higher doses than normal. Some patients with skin disorders required 40,000 IU daily to correct their deficiencies. Considering that most vitamin D supplements are 400 IU, this dose is incredibly high. But it worked for them. Their skin and their immune health improved without any side effects. Therefore, please work with a functional or integrative professional to test and correct your vitamin D levels as necessary.

Healthy Fats

Healthy skin requires healthy fats, otherwise known as lipids. Remember, when I covered the formation of healthy skin, lipids (fats) were one of the substances carried up through the layers of the skin. Then, when the cells collapse in the final stratum corneum layer, the lipids spill out and provide a water-proof coating around the cells to help minimise water evaporation and the ingress of undesirable substances.

Omega-3 fats are essential for the health of our skin and brain, particularly eicosapentaenoic acid (EPA) and docosahexaenoic acid (DHA) from fish, krill, or marine algae. Unfortunately, some older strict vegans who have not taken omega-3 supplements have developed signs of neurodegenerative diseases due to the impact of essential fatty acid deficiency on their brains. Conversely, some children with attention deficit disorders have shown improvement after supplementing their diets with omega-3 fats. Additionally, essential fatty acid deficiency can lead to dry skin disorders with scaly rashes like eczema, poor wound healing, greying hair, increased susceptibility to infections, and difficulty concentrating.

Marine sources of omega-3 fatty acids have been shown to reduce inflammatory reactions by inhibiting the production of prostaglandins, similar to the effects exerted by ginger root. Scientists investigated krill oil extracted from zooplankton crustaceans in the Antarctic region due to its anti-inflammatory effects in patients with cardiovascular and rheumatoid arthritis. These conditions (in addition to other inflammatory conditions) lead to elevated levels of inflammatory markers in the blood called C-reactive proteins. The higher the level of inflammation in a person's body, the higher the level of C-reaction proteins observed in their blood. In a randomised, placebo-controlled, double-blind trial, treatment with krill oil (300 mg daily) significantly reduced both the C-reactive protein levels and the arthritic symptoms such as joint pain, stiffness, and functional impairment. (68) Although this particular study was sponsored by the manufacturer of the krill oil brand used, many other studies are extolling the virtues of supplementing omega-3 fats to help with chronic inflammatory conditions such as eczema. In one study involving pregnant women, fish consumption throughout their pregnancies was recorded, and researchers assessed the correlation with eczema development in their infants. Those infants born to women with the highest intake of eicosapentaenoic acid and docosahexaenoic acid from oily fish showed a clear reduction in their risk of eczema development. (93)

Eicosapentaenoic acid and docosahexaenoic acid oils elicit an anti-inflammatory effect on the immune system and assist in wound healing in the skin. Both of these are welcome additions when trying to disengage eczema's inflammatory cycles. If you do not want to take fish oil supplements, you can get marine algae supplements that are also effective.

Soybeans and nuts also have a high content of unsaturated plant forms of omega-3 fatty acids and can also be a valuable dietary source of healthy fats. Still, care must be taken by those with eczema as these are two of the most common allergens. It would be best if you also sourced organic producers as nuts, especially soya, are often sprayed with pesticides and are genetically modified. Other good fat sources are avocados, coconut oil, flax seeds, chia seeds, and olive oil.

Zinc

Zinc is a mineral nutrient known to be vital for skin health. It is involved in numerous processes, including activating skin hormones, regulating skin inflammation, and regenerating skin cells. Several proteins in the human body need to bind with zinc to conduct their biological activities. The extent to which these processes can occur is linked directly to zinc concentration in the body and its availability to the cells. Zinc deficiency has been shown to lead to dermatitis, decreased immune function, and slow wound healing. It is one of the minerals that are commonly deficient in eczema patients. (76) Zinc binds to toxic metals and assists in excreting them from the body; therefore, a deficiency can result in inefficient toxin removal and the build-up of heavy metals in the body. Toxicity is also implicated in eczema development and severity, which we look at in more detail in Chapter 12.

The greatest food sources of zinc are crab and lobster, followed by red meat, poultry, beans, and legumes. Unfortunately, most non-meat sources of zinc are found in food which can be problematic for those with atopic conditions. These sources include eggs, dairy, nuts, and seeds, common eczema flare triggers. Therefore, eczema sufferers must carefully consider planning adequate dietary intake from safe sources or taking a trusted supplement. (I say 'trusted' because many supplements can have fillers and undesirable ingredients added.)

Vitamin C

In a clinical study, eczema patients were seen to have deficient antioxidant levels, particularly of vitamins A, C, and E, which would compound the issue of oxidative stress as being low in these antioxidants reduces the inability to correct oxidation. (76)

Vitamin C is a powerful natural antihistamine that can reduce allergic tendencies and serum histamine levels, which is an excellent tool for anyone suffering from atopic diseases. It is also a highly effective antioxidant, helping to clear free radicals from the body and minimise the damage from oxidation.

Vitamin C is also vital for collagen production, which is crucial for the integrity of our skin. It is also essential for immune function and wound repair. Deficiency symptoms include easy bruising, bleeding gums, frequent nose bleeds, poor wound healing, decreased ability to fight infections, muscle and joint pains, and dry skin.

Unlike many other animals, humans cannot store vitamin C. Therefore, we must obtain it daily from the diet. Furthermore, it only lasts in the body for around 3-4 hours; thus, we should eat a variety of fresh fruits throughout the day to give us regular supplies of vitamin C. It is present in vegetables, too but is destroyed by cooking, so salads are a good option for vegetable sources.

Making fresh juices and smoothies are also effective ways to increase your vitamin C intake. For example, squeezing fresh lemon juice into your drinking water 3-4 times a day is a great way to improve both your vitamin C and bioflavonoid intake. Although the recommended vitamin C intake is around 50 mg daily, this is woefully inadequate for those with chronic inflammatory diseases such as eczema. I have already spoken of the merits of supplementing with high dose vitamin C, and I would repeat my recommendation that you read: '**Vitamin C: The Real Story**' by Steve Hickey, PhD, and Andrew W. Saul, PhD.

Vitamin E

Vitamin E is another potent antioxidant but with the added ability to reduce serum IgE levels in atopic patients. It is already known to elicit protective effects against common health problems such as heart disease, cataracts, cancer, and stroke when taken at high enough levels.

The natural alpha-tocopherol form of vitamin E prevents oxidative stress due to free radicals on cell membranes. It is involved in the activation of some molecules and enzymes in immune and inflammatory cells. It protects the outer membranes of your macrophage immune cells against oxidative damage and reduces the production of prostaglandins by the immune system. Serum IgE levels have been reduced by vitamin E supplementation, even at low doses of just 400 mg a day, with no side effects. (42) Interestingly, for eczema patients, vitamin E is also necessary for making keratin, which is essential for producing healthy keratinocyte skin cells. (20)

Obtaining sufficient vitamin E from dietary sources can be problematic for eczema patients and those who have developed atopic conditions. The highest sources are found primarily in common allergen foods such as wheatgerm, nuts, seeds and their oils, and oily fish. Avocados also have high amounts of vitamin E. Although this is not one of the most common allergens, sensitisation to avocados has been rising, perhaps due to the chemicals used to farm non-organic varieties.

Vitamin A

From an eczema point of view, vitamin A is a fascinating nutrient. In laboratory tests, vitamin A deficient mice showed significantly more mast cells accumulating in their eczema skin lesions, more severe Th2-mediated inflammation, higher circulating blood levels of both IgG1 and IgE antibodies, increased IL-4 and IL-13 inflammatory cytokines, and a reduced Th1 immune response. Thus, vitamin A deficiency directly exacerbates eczema by increasing Th2-mediated inflammation and mast cell activation. Therapeutic vitamin A supplementation can rescue the vitamin A deficient type of atopic dermatitis, and scientists have considered that it may provide a new strategy for future prevention or treatment of atopic dermatitis in general. (38) Vitamin A deficiency is also linked to keratin deficiency and keratosis pilaris, another skin condition associated with filaggrin deficiency. (1) Vitamin A is vital for immune health and is rapidly depleted from the liver during illness. A study published in 1987 showed that supplementation reduced death and severe complications from childhood illnesses such as measles and chicken pox when given in extremely high doses (one single dose of 200,000 IU). (84)

Vitamin A is another fat-soluble vitamin that can become toxic if taken to excess; therefore, I reiterate the importance of working with a functional or integrative professional qualified to assess your nutritional status and prescribe remedial treatments. Although the body can convert beta-carotene from green and orange plants into vitamin A, not everyone does this efficiently. A study by the World Health Organization stated that six times more beta-carotene must be ingested to obtain the same therapeutic effects as the more readily absorbable form called retinol. (85) However, beta-carotene supplementation has been implicated with an increased risk of cancer development, so taking six times the dose to achieve the therapeutic levels of retinol may well be counterproductive. The form used in the eczema studies was the retinol type, which is derived only from animal sources such as liver, oily fish, eggs, cheese, and butter. It is easy to become deficient in vitamin A if you are allergic to dairy products and eggs, as many eczema patients are, and even more so if you do not like the taste of liver or fish.

Biotin

Biotin is one of the B vitamins and is another nutrient necessary for making keratin. It is found predominantly in liver, although there are smaller amounts in fish, whole grains, nuts, and broccoli. Biotin deficiencies lead to thinning hair and dermatitis-type rashes around the eyes, nose, and mouth. (20) The *Bifidobacterium* family of probiotics in the gut microbiome help to produce biotin; therefore, having depleted gut colonies of *Bifidobacterium* will impact your ability to produce and absorb biotin.

Niacin

Niacin, otherwise known as vitamin B3, is vital for producing the co-enzyme nicotinamide adenine dinucleotide (NAD), which is required for over four hundred enzymes reactions to be performed effectively, including enzyme reactions that control gene expressions and cellular communication. (67) It also has a role in repairing DNA and functions as an antioxidant. Niacin deficiency leads to poor circulation, increased allergic nature, mouth ulcers, dermatitis-type rashes, and neurological disorders such as bipolar disorder and depression. A lack of niacin also causes cells to hold increased amounts of histamine, which means there is more to release during allergic reactions. Be careful if you take niacin supplements, as its ability to release histamine from cells can cause a rather intense flushing effect. This can cause a sensation of heat, red flushing, prickling in the skin, and in extreme cases, a drop in blood pressure. It can be quite alarming if you experience an intense flush, especially if you were not forewarned. Some people even assumed they were having an allergic reaction to the niacin and attended the hospital. I can understand why, as I once enthusiastically took a large dose of niacin and consequently turned purple. My children were fascinated. It is an amusing memory now, but if I had not known about the flushing effects, I think I would have been quite scared too. However, knowing what was happening, I was able to stay calm and wait for it to pass. Niacinamide is an alternative version of vitamin B3 that does not cause flushing and may be preferable if you are prescribed B3 to treat a deficiency. Liver, fish, beef, chicken, and turkey are good food sources of niacin. Legumes, nuts, and seeds also provide smaller amounts, but they are less readily absorbed as they are bound by anti-nutrient compounds naturally present in these foods. Consequently, only around 30% of the available niacin in plant foods is absorbed. (67) If you have psoriasis in addition to eczema, you need to be careful regarding supplementing with niacin. Although it commonly helps with eczema, it can be problematic for people with psoriasis and can increase its severity in some patients. So seek professional advice if this applies to you.

Vitamin B12

Vitamin B12 is essential as it is involved in the metabolism of every cell in the human body and is also used to synthesise essential fatty acids such as omega-3 oils from fish. In addition, it is involved in the creation and regulation of DNA and is crucial for correct brain and nerve function and the formation of red blood cells. Vitamin B12 deficiency causes the red blood cells to become enlarged and may also die earlier than normal. Consequently, oxygen-carrying capacity depletes, leading to shortness of breath and fatigue. These symptoms do not always occur though, and many people experience other less obvious signs of deficiency, such as depression, swelling of the tongue, frequent pins and needles, deteriorating eyesight, brain fog, and constipation. Vitamin B12 deficiency is also commonly seen in people with hypothyroidism, which can also exhibit many of the same symptoms as vitamin B12 deficiency.

Vitamin B12 can be obtained readily from a healthy diet. The most significant sources are meat products and fish, especially lamb liver and steak, sardines, tuna, trout, and salmon. However, if there is damage to the gut lining, there may be malabsorption issues, which could affect the ability to utilise the vitamin B12 in their diet. In such cases, sublingual vitamin B12 supplements, which are absorbed under the tongue, will be a better option. I believe sub-lingual vitamin B12 is a safer option than injections as I am dubious about the integrity and full disclosure of injection ingredients in our current environment.

Although vitamin B12 has not been exhaustively studied for eczema, there does appear to be a link between vitamin B12 deficiency and the severity of atopic dermatitis; some patients have even seen symptoms improve with vitamin B12 supplementation. Vitamin B12 has a complex relationship with the skin; either deficiencies or excess can cause changes in the skin and tongue. Therefore, it is advisable to check your vitamin B12 status. Chronic stress can also deplete the body of vitamin B12, and eczema patients have been shown to have higher stress responses and anxiety levels due to their chronic discomfort and sleep deprivation. Hence, supplementation may be beneficial. Sublingual forms that can be absorbed under the tongue can often be more effective than a tablet, as having gut dysbiosis or inflammation can impair the absorption of vitamin B12 from the gut. Studies have shown that 5000 mcg of the sublingual supplement daily raises blood levels of vitamin B12 to an equivalent of that achieved by 1000 mcg of injected vitamin B12.

Pyridoxine Vitamin B6

Pyridoxine is another one of the B vitamins involved in maintaining our immune health. It is also essential for processing amino acids, red blood cell formation, and proper functioning of the nervous system, amongst many other functions. A deficiency of vitamin B6 can exhibit dermatitis-type rashes, anaemia, depression, nerve damage, and an increased risk of heart disease. Vitamin B6 is another vitamin that can be harmful if taken to excess, as toxic levels can cause nerve damage similar to that seen in deficiency.

The highest quantities of vitamin B6 in the diet are found in salmon and meat; sweet potatoes, potatoes, and bananas also have relatively high amounts. In addition, most multivitamins will contain vitamin B6.

Electrolytes

One interesting study showed that every single eczema sufferer was seen to be abnormally low in the electrolytes, calcium, potassium, and sodium. These minerals are all essential for proper cellular function and detoxification. Deficiencies in them will contribute to oxidative stress and toxic overload, increasing inflammation. (76) I will talk more about oxidative stress in the next chapter, 'The Stress Connection', but it is worth checking your electrolyte levels. The best source of electrolytes for supplementation is natural coconut water, which according to the website nutrieats.com has a similar electrolyte ratio to healthy human blood. It is also devoid of artificial additives and added sugar, making it a much healthier choice than commercially produced substitutes.

TUDCA

The final supplement I want to discuss is TUDCA, which is short for Tauroursodeoxychloric acid. TUDCA is a bile salt supplement that has numerous health benefits, such as increasing the absorption rate of vitamin D, stimulating bile production and flow, reducing liver in-flammation, improving insulin resistance, helping to repair leaky gut, aiding in the restoration of the gut microbiome, improving cognitive performance, reducing anxiety and depression, and lowering the levels of circulating inflammatory cytokines. As we have seen that many of these issues are implicated or somehow involved in the eczema cycles, TUDCA is an extremely promising addition to your supplement regime. Further benefits of supplementing with TUDCA are still being discovered.

The Bitter Side of Sweet

No chapter on healthy nutrition and diet would be complete without a section on the impact of sugar. If you have a sweet tooth, this section may be a bitter reading experience for you. I make no apology though. You really do need to know what you do to yourself when you eat refined sugar, especially concerning how it impacts your skin.

When we eat, our body will convert the sugars in our food to glucose, which is then taken up by our cells and used as energy. Sugar itself is not the enemy if used wisely, but refined sugar or excess sugar is. Your body already knows that excess sugar is toxic. That is why we have our insulin mechanism to regulate blood sugar levels and prevent them from rising too high. Insulin is a hormone produced by cells in the pancreas when glucose levels rise in the blood after eating. It enables the cells to take up the glucose, which is used either for energy or stored as fat for later use if it is currently surplus to requirements. People with diabetes who cannot produce or respond to insulin must check their blood sugar levels regularly. Elevated glucose in the blood is known to cause serious health consequences including diabetic coma, nerve damage, blindness, and even death. While you may think that this does not apply to you if you do not have diabetes, sugar also causes other insidious effects that have some quite drastic detrimental impacts on skin formation, immune function, fungal infections, allergic nature, the microbiome, and stress, all of which are involved in eczema.

The typical guideline from health advisers is that adults should not consume more than six teaspoons of sugar daily, and a child's intake should be below three teaspoons. Unfortunately, this is still too high. However, most people who consume the standard Westernized diet will eat far more than this, even if they do not actively eat sweets and candies. This is because refined sugar is added to a huge variety of food products, often as different names that consumers do not recognise as sugar. According to an article published by John Hopkins Medicine, there are over 60 different names for sugar. Added sugars will usually (but not always) contain one of three clues in their name: syrup, sugar, or words ending in 'ose', such as fructose and glucose. Honey, agave, concentrated fruit juice, and fruit nectar are other ingredients that simply mean 'added sugar'.

Do you see why it is so easy to far exceed the recommended sugar limit without even trying? Even when we avoid eating candies, we can inadvertently consume high quantities of these ingredients in sauces, condiments, ready-made meals, cereals, bread, and a host of refined man-made foods. Then there are other items we know are laden with sugar, but many people still buy them anyway because they are unknowingly addicted to them. For example, one small 8 oz serving of lemonade can contain six teaspoons of sugar. A 330 ml soda can contains eight teaspoons, each cookie contains one teaspoon, and a slice of cake contains four teaspoons. These are without mentioning the high amounts of sugar in condiments such as ketchup, barbecue sauce, and seasonings like teriyaki. In addition, many people are unaware that different foods convert to glucose at varying speeds in the body. This is called the glycemic index of the food. Therefore, even if they do not contain refined sugar, some food items cause rapid blood sugar rises because they are converted so quickly to glucose. The most common culprits are food items that have been refined and made into 'white' versions, such as white bread, white pasta, and white rice. 'White' food items have had the outer husk removed, which contains the fibre and minerals. Fibre is harder for the body to break down, which delays the release of sugars from the food. If we eat high glycemic foods (the ones that release sugars rapidly) throughout the day, our blood sugar will spike each time we eat them. Then, our pancreas will be forced to release insulin to remove the excess sugar by directing the cells to take up the glucose. The insulin release can then cause the sugar levels to reduce below the desired level, which can cause sugar cravings and irritability. Off we go to grab another sugary snack and the rollercoaster ride repeats itself throughout the day, leaving us feeling constantly exhausted, battling reoccurring headaches, and fighting brain fog. Living with the constant barrage of excess sugar and the resulting flood of insulin can cause the pancreas to become less efficient at producing insulin and the cells to become less responsive over time to the insulin produced, leading to a diagnosis of type 2 diabetes. Low sugar levels also increase cortisol and stress hormones. As these are released into the bloodstream, the body is placed on high alert, in 'fight or flight' mode. Stress suppresses digestion, healing, immune function, and healthy sleep, all of which impact eczema risk and severity. The next chapter is a deep dive into how stress affects eczema.

Sugar also feeds yeast, which eczema sufferers can already find challenging to keep under control. As mentioned previously, eczema sufferers typically display higher levels of yeast colonisation on their skin than non-eczema sufferers. In addition, a diet overly high in sugar encourages an overpopulation of yeast microbes in the gut. These critters can cause sugar cravings, irritability, anxiety, and a host of other health problems by contributing to gut and skin dysbiosis. Feeding yeast can lead directly to eczema flare-ups. I have worked with people and helped them discover that they could eliminate all their eczema flares if they eliminated sugar from their diet. This may also be because sugar depresses the immune system, particularly macrophage activity. Glucose, having a very similar molecular structure to vitamin C, can be taken up by the ascorbate receptors on the cells. Still, instead of supercharging them as vitamin C would do, it makes the cells lethargic and inefficient for up to seven hours. This allows the pathogenic bacterium, including *Staphylococcus*, to increase their colonisation unhindered, thus increasing the thymic stromal lymphopoietin cycle I spoke of previously and the resulting inflammation.

Furthermore, high glucose levels in the blood encourage higher levels of histamine, which cause itching, redness, and irritation in the skin. Sugar clearly is not an essential nutrient and has many adverse health implications. You will benefit significantly from reducing your intake.

Concluding Nutrition

Nutrition is a complex study, and nutritional status requires personal assessment and testing. Various tests can highlight deficiencies; hair and urine tests can be more accurate at detecting deficiencies as they show the amount of nutrients that have been absorbed by our cells rather than those flowing freely in the bloodstream. Just because we eat something, it does not mean our gut absorbs it well, and just because we have it in our bloodstream, it does not mean our cells can utilise it effectively. I am not recommending you go out and buy supplements for all the possible nutritional deficiencies I have listed. The purpose of this list is to give you guidance on what nutritional deficiencies to test for. I highly recommend working with a functional or integrative professional to assess your individual nutritional deficiencies and to take supplements as required to correct them.

One of the best ways to test for nutritional deficiencies is to have a hair analysis. This involves taking a sample of your recent hair growth near the scalp. Remember how I said you are what you absorb, not what you eat? Your hair more accurately shows what you have absorbed, which is why it is often used to test for illicit drug use. Many functional and integrative medicine professionals can provide this test, which I highly recommend. However, although I do recommend taking supplements to provide extra support to your body, supplements are supplements, meaning 'in addition to'. They are designed to supplement your diet, not to be taken instead of a healthy diet. So, yes, get your nutritional status checked, but please do not take supplements and then just eat junk. We need to nurture our bodies through our diet and then supplement the things our body needs for extra support, as necessary.

When we look at the eczema spider web now, we have learnt that diet and nutritional status directly affect our skin health as there are numerous nutritional deficiencies that can cause a dry dysfunctional skin barrier and dermatitis-type rash, even in people who do not have any genetic mutations predisposing them to eczema. In addition, our diet and nutritional profile also affect our gut health and microbiome balance, our DNA expression for disease risks and protein manufacture, our immune health, our detoxing ability, and our allergic susceptibility. Furthermore, deficiencies also increase stress levels in the body.

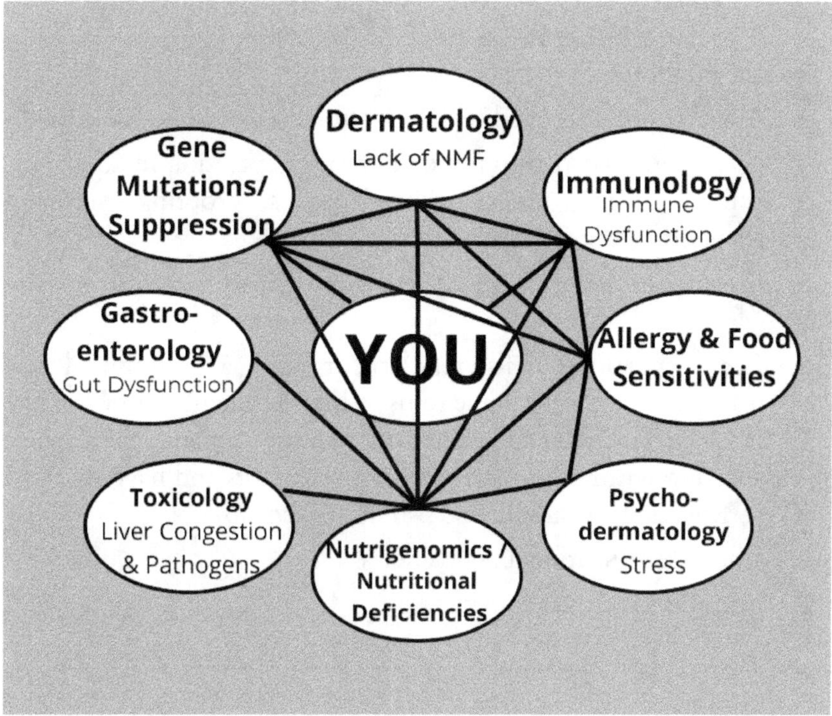

Next, we will look at the microbiome in more detail and consider how the state of our microflora impacts our health. This is a real eye-opener!

Here are your action points for this chapter.

Action points

1. Increase your plant food intake. Remember to eat something raw with every meal. Add as many vegetables as possible to salads, smoothies, raw juices, stews, casseroles, and soups.

2. Eat rainbows.

3. Avoid genetically modified, bioengineered, or transgenic foods.

4. Learn about correct (traditional) food preparation methods, including cleaning meat, soaking legumes, sprouting seeds, and fermenting vegetables.

5. Incorporate prebiotic foods into your diet to feed your gut organisms.

6. Consider eating oily fish regularly or taking a clean fish oil supplement. Personally, I like to use a brand called Eskimo 3. They produce both adult and child Omega 3 supplements, are 3rd party tested to ensure they are free from pollutants and have received certification for sustainable fishing methods.

7. Check for nutritional deficiencies.

8. Minimise your sugar intake.

10

The Rainforest Within

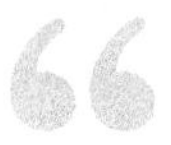

All disease begins in the gut."

Hippocrates

Sprawling across Brazil and seven other countries in the South American continent is the Amazon rainforest. Covering over 7 million km² of land, it makes up over half of the remaining rainforest area worldwide. According to Wikipedia, 10% of all known species live in the Amazon rainforest, with 20% of all bird and fish species, 40,000 different plant types, and 2.5 million insect species. It hosts the most extensive collection of species in the world, with an unparalleled biodiversity of plants. To date, an estimated 438,000 species of plants in the region have been registered as having particular economic or social interests, with more species still being discovered. What a fascinating place!

The Amazon is also home to numerous creatures that can pose a threat to humans. For example, in the Amazon River, you could encounter piranhas and electric eels, whilst on land, there are black caimans, jaguars, cougars, anacondas, poison dart frogs, vampire bats carrying rabies, numerous parasites, and of course, mosquitoes that carry and transmit malaria, yellow fever, and dengue fever. However, left to its own devices and without human interference, it does an outstanding job of keeping its biodiversity under control. Each species has its own contribution to make to the ecological system, which manages its own diversity, keeping the correct proportions of species to maintain equilibrium or balance.

The winds carry copious amounts of Sahara dust across the Atlantic to the South American region every year. Although much of it falls into the sea, still enough reaches South America and the Caribbean to impact the air quality. In Trinidad and Tobago, we can be severely affected by it in the dry season, even to the point of being advised that it is unhealthy to be outside sometimes. The Northern range mountains that can be seen for miles disappear entirely under a cloud of dust and cannot be seen until you are almost upon them. However, those same Sahara dust plumes that cause air quality problems for the residents of Trinidad and Tobago also provide great fertilising benefits for the Amazon. Around 28 million tons of dust fall over the Amazon basin, over 22 million of which consists of phosphorous, which is particularly important for plant growth and helps keep the Amazon lush and green. Numerous cycles replenish the water and nutrients in the soil to keep the land fertile. The density of the plants and the vast land area covered by the Amazon enable it to function as a massive carbon sink, absorbing 2 billion tons of carbon dioxide gas every year. The Amazon is vital to maintaining the health of our planet.

Sadly, human ignorance and greed have destroyed much of the Amazon rainforest. By 2020, over 20% (more than 587,000 km^2) had been destroyed, the majority for temporary farming land. In addition, more than 200,000 acres are burned every day. This leads me to ask two questions:

1. What effects do you think the destruction of the Amazon will have on the remaining ecosystem of the jungle and the world at large?
2. Why has this got anything to do with healing eczema?

The answer to the first question is quite frightening. According to rain-tree.com, researchers have studied less than 1% of the millions of species in the Amazon. Yet, as the Amazon is destroyed, scientists estimate that 137 species of plants and animals are lost every single day. Whole species are driven to extinction at local levels and some to global extinction. We have yet to discover the roles these species have in maintaining the health of the ecosystem and planet. Hence, we have yet to realise the full extent of the damage we have caused by our ignorance and greed.

The answer to the second question is that you have your own personal 'rainforest' living inside you, which, left to its own devices and allowed to live in its unadulterated state, would function in a beautiful equilibrium, keeping you healthy and balanced. But just as the Amazon has been disturbed and much of it destroyed by our stupidity masked in the veil of progress, so has the 'rainforest' inside you. Whole species have been driven to extinction at our local level, yet we still have not discovered all the species within us or learned of all their roles in maintaining the health of our bodies. Just as some are starting to wake up and realise that damage to the Amazon will bring lasting consequences to our planet, people are also waking up to the implications of the damage we are causing to our precious microbiome and the lasting consequences to our health. With that said, let me introduce you to your "Mighty Microbiome: The Rainforest Within."

The Mighty Microbiome

The microbiome is the collective name given to all the bacteria, fungi, archaea, and viruses that live on us and in us. Together, they weigh around 2 kg in an adult, yet we have about 39 trillion microbial cells in our body, which means the microbial cells outnumber our own. Although the largest microbiome community occupies your gut, you have many varied and distinct microbiome communities all over your body, internally and externally. For example, the colony of microbes that reside in your armpit has a different composition to that which resides in your mouth, which is different again to that which populates your feet and that which occupies your gut. Likewise, your hands have their own distinct microbiome and so do your lungs.

The microbiome in our gut is now known to have an essential role in the digestion and absorption of nutrients from our food. However, the role of the complete microbiome is so much more than this. It includes detoxifying our cells and organs, breaking down and eliminating heavy metals and toxic chemicals, controlling our immune system, keeping pathogenic bacterial populations in check, re-enforcing the mucosal lining of the gastrointestinal tract, and producing the neurotransmitters required for effective brain function. It even has a vital role in hormone regulation. Indeed, the microbiome is pretty much responsible for keeping us alive. So, where do we get all these microbes from?

Well, your microbiome is inherited primarily from your mother. It is the one inherited feature that your mother naturally has a far greater input than your father, simply because she was the one who carried you and gave birth to you. In the last three weeks before birth, the microbiome in the mother's birth canal changes to provide the perfect mix of microbes to populate the body of the new infant as they pass through and emerge into the world. These microbes provide our earliest immune system along with all the other roles they play. Indeed, a 2014 study found that infants born by cesarean section had a higher risk of developing atopy, including allergies and eczema. Furthermore, the risk was also increased for vaginally born babies whose mothers had taken antibiotics at any time during pregnancy. (72) This is because an infant who either does not pass through the birth canal (or who passes through one that has been decimated of microbes due to the mother's antibiotic exposure) does not get populated with all the healthy microbes that should have provided their first microbiome community.

When a baby breastfeeds, for the first two days, they do not receive milk but instead colostrum. This high-calorie fluid is full of probiotics, prebiotics, and antibodies from the mother's immune system. The pre-and probiotics prepare the infant's gastrointestinal tract to receive and be able to digest the mother's milk, which then provides the perfect nutrition for the developing infant. Breast milk also contains the mother's IgA antibodies, which populate the infant's gut and help to provide healthy tolerance to food proteins. A study published in 1936 examined over 20,000 infants to determine if there was a correlation between feeding breast milk or formula milk and the development of eczema. They concluded that feeding infants with a combination of breast and formula milk had doubled risk of developing eczema and formula feeding alone created a seven-fold risk of developing eczema compared to breastfeeding alone. (71) This was long before anyone realised the importance of the microbiome and how natural birth and breastfeeding help to establish a healthy gut microflora. The purpose of my sharing this information is not to condemn anyone for not giving birth vaginally or for not breastfeeding. There are many reasons why either may not be possible. My intention is merely to inform you of the discoveries that have been made scientifically to enable you to gain awareness of probable root causes for your own or your child's eczema.

The microbes that live inside us and on us are termed either pathogenic or commensurate. Pathogenic microbes would be harmful to us if they were over-populated, whereas commensurate microbes are typically viewed as friendly. However, any microbe that invades into a different area to which it belongs would not be welcome and can cause health problems, much like the jaguar leaving the Amazon rainforest and entering a village. Generally, left to its own devices, our microbiome does a great job of maintaining its own equilibrium, ensuring the pathogenic organisms are kept in check by the commensurate ones. Collectively, we live in what is called a symbiotic relationship, meaning that we help each other and are interdependent on one another. We give the microbes a home and food to eat, and they help to look after us. However, if you compare the amount of DNA in them and the amount of DNA in us, their DNA outnumbers ours. Thus, it leads us to wonder who is really helping who the most.

You may be wondering what these organisms do and why they are so important. I will run through some of their essential roles. Remember, we still have yet to discover every organism and everything they are responsible for, so the depth of this knowledge will continue to grow as more discoveries are made.

In Digesting Food

The organisms in our gut create bacterial pathways that help us digest our food and utilise the nutrients, which include vitamins, minerals, complex carbohydrates, proteins, and fats. (5) We often think that food is digested by stomach acid and enzymes; however, our microbes digest more of our food than we do. This is because we do not possess all the enzymes needed to digest all the foods we should eat, but microbes do (I am not talking about junk food here, but real food). For example, humans only possess 17 enzymes capable of breaking down and digesting carbohydrates into absorbable matter. If we were to exist with only these 17 enzymes, we would be severely restricted in the diversity of carbohydrate-based foods we could eat as we would only be able to digest a limited variety of them. In contrast, a healthy microbiome possesses over 16,000 carbohydrate-specific enzymes. Thus, our microbes digest a vast array of carbohydrates for us and release beneficial compounds from them through our gut lining into our bodies. In addition, certain microbe colonies also ferment amino acids, which is vital for protein digestion and absorption. (46) Decimating our gut microbes through years of antibiotic use in our own and previous generations will wipe out colonies of microbiota, including their specific carbohydrate-digesting abilities. This will result in the inability to digest certain carbohydrate foods and consequently lead to food intolerances due to reduced digestive capability and deficiencies in the beneficial healing compounds provided by those foods.

One example that is relevant to eczema is histidine. Histidine-deficient diets have been shown to result in an eczematous rash in infants and adults, as histidine directly impacts the quality of the skin barrier. (1, 4) Histidine is also responsible for maintaining the myelin sheath around nerve cells and joints; thus, a deficiency can also lead to arthritis. (9) There is also a possible link between histidine deficiency and multiple sclerosis.

We already spoke of the necessity of histidine in producing healthy skin and how dietary supplementation improves the skin's barrier function quite dramatically. Now we are taking it deeper and discovering another reason why low histidine is often a problem for eczema patients. A histidine deficiency can also be caused by low levels of histidine-synthesising gut microbes, which results in the inability to utilise the histidine consumed in the diet effectively. Certain microbes help break down the carnosine in meat to release the free (useable) form of histidine. Minimal carnosine activity by gut microbes leads to a reduced ability to release the free form of histidine from the carnosine in the sources we consume. (1) Carnosine is found chiefly in meat which is why the word starts with a derivative of 'carni' (the Latin word for 'flesh') as in 'carnivore'. There are also trace amounts in eggs and dairy produce. The most significant sources of carnosine in our diet are from muscle meats. The stronger the muscle, the greater the carnosine content. We have already established the importance of histidine to people with eczema. This inability to release and utilise the histidine from the carnosine in meat is a further cause of a potential histidine deficiency in addition to those caused by the gene mutations we spoke of in Chapter 6. It also would explain why eczema sufferers often fare better on a diet containing more meat than those with clear skin. It is similar to the orthomolecular medicine model of prescribing mega doses of nutrients where damage to the gut or gut dysbiosis leads to a reduced ability to absorb these nutrients at 'normal' amounts.

You will recall how I discussed histidine supplementation to help alleviate a histidine deficiency in people with eczema. L-histidine is an amino acid known to be synthesised inefficiently by humans because we have low levels of histidine synthesising gut microflora and minimal carnosine activity. (If we had these, they would help us release the free form of L-histidine from the carnosine in meat.) Therefore, if we deplete our microbes any further by antibiotic use and other microbiome killers, we can quickly become histidine deficient, even if there is sufficient consumption in the diet. If you couple microbial depletion with a gene mutation for filaggrin, the odds are stacked against you for eczema development. As stated in "Feeding Filaggrin: Effects of L-Histidine Supplementation in Atopic Dermatitis", published in 2017:

"Histidine deficiency is especially detrimental if a genetic predisposition exists for filaggrin loss of function mutations on the epidermal differentiation complex portion of chromosome 1." (1)

Another role of gut microbes is to break down and ferment complex carbohydrate foods, enabling us to absorb their nutrients. As a direct result of this fermentation process, the microbes release substances called short-chain fatty acids, which are essential for our gut and brain health. For example, butyrate is produced by certain microbes when they ferment complex carbohydrates from foods such as root vegetables. It is vital for repairing the gut lining, re-enforcing the mucosal barrier, and helping to keep the pathogenic bacterium from invading out of the gut lining and into the surrounding tissues (commonly known as leaky gut). Lacking these microbes reduces the ability to digest certain carbohydrates, resulting in food intolerances and the development of irritable bowel syndrome-type symptoms.

The microbes are also responsible for helping to break down proteins into their amino acids. As stated previously, amino acids are the building blocks of virtually everything made in the body, from molecules to enzymes, which are required for maintenance and repair tasks. They are like the minuscule Lego structures I mentioned before. You eat protein in one form, say meat, and your body breaks it down into amino acids, the tiniest Lego bricks, and then rebuilds them according to what it needs to function optimally. If your microbe colonies are depleted, they cannot help you to break down and absorb the proteins. Consequently, you will not have the amino acids you need to perform the necessary functions in your body. Your health will then start to suffer, and you will develop dis-ease.

The digestion of one particular amino acid, called arginine, by gut microbes leads to three essential polyamines. (Polyamines are compounds with two or more amino groups joined together. Poly means many, and Amin is derived from amino acid.) The polyamines in question are called agmatine, putrescine, and spermine, all of which improve the integrity of the gut by various means, including increasing the expression of tight junction proteins, encouraging healing of the gut lining, and increasing the secretion of gastrointestinal mucus. Interestingly, putrescine and spermine can also suppress the production of pro-inflammatory cytokines, such as IL-6 and TNF-α. Arginine can additionally be converted to glutamate, from which we produce gamma-aminobutyric acid (GABA). Gamma-aminobutyric acid is a critical neurotransmitter for the central nervous system. Deficiencies in gamma-aminobutyric acid are linked to the development of depression and anxiety, which affects those suffering from eczema more commonly than those who do not. (45) GABA can additionally regulate the proliferation of helper T cells and can therefore modulate the immune system responses. Interestingly, chronic inflammation in the gastrointestinal tract was reported to induce anxiety in mice. In addition, depression and anxiety sufferers have been found to have co-existing gastrointestinal disorders, including irritable bowel syndrome.

Another microbe colony relevant to eczema is *Bifidobacterium*, which produces biotin; this is required by the body to effectively make the keratin needed in the keratinocyte skin cells. (20) If the gut microbes are depleted, a keratin deficiency may also occur, affecting the skin barrier's structural integrity, even without any genetic mutations for keratin production.

Another research paper published in 2009 titled: "Eczema Genetics: Current state of knowledge and future goals" states:

"Extensive lack of amino acid fermenting bacterium such as *Clostridium* clusters, *Bacillus, Lactobacillus, Streptococcus* groups, and *Proteobacterium* have been shown to lead to impaired protein digestion and subsequent amino acid absorption in the gastrointestinal tract." (9)

Therefore, if we decimate our microbial colonies, we no longer possess the means to digest the foods we eat and will not have enough amino acids or other nutrients to absorb and utilise. Consequently, even if you eat well, you may still develop malnutrition-related diseases.

A group of scientists conducted tests on infants with microbiome dysbiosis to analyse the effects of dysbiosis on their digestion. Their findings confirmed that having depleted microbial communities and species detrimentally affected digestive capabilities. However, interestingly, the results showed that gut dysbiosis causes even more expansive digestive dysfunction than the scientists had predicted. The deficiencies involved a wide range of lipids (fats), amino acids, carbohydrates, peptides, xenobiotics, nucleotides, vitamins, and energy metabolism pathways. (5) Infants with a disturbed gut microbiome will be unable to digest and absorb all the required nutrients, even those in their mother's milk. As a result, their health will suffer. This can also present as food intolerances and allergic tendencies in older infants who are weaned and other children. However, although this study was conducted with infants, it is relevant for adults too. Gut dysbiosis will seriously impact your ability to digest the food you eat and, consequently, nutrient absorption.

The above research corroborates what I frequently explain to eczema sufferers. To say, "We are what we eat", is simply not true. It is far more accurate to say, "We are what we absorb." It also explains why so many people in developed countries suffer diseases of malnutrition even though they have an abundance of food available. A lot of so-called food in the Western world is simply junk devoid of nutrients. When we do eat real food, we may no longer be able to digest it due to the depletion of microbe populations. The microbial diversity of your gut directly reflects the variety of plant foods in your diet. Consequently, if we hardly ever eat real plant food in its natural state, the colonies that should be there to digest those foods will die off. These microbes regulate our hormones, help to break down toxins and help us digest our vitamins, minerals, and healthy fats. Thus, a deficiency of these colonies can mean we end up nutritionally deficient even if we eat a healthy diet. I will say this again as it is worth repeating, "You are what you absorb" is far more accurate than "You are what you eat."

Deficiencies can cause a whole host of health issues, not just in the realm of eczema. However, your vitamin needs do not depend on the recommended daily allowance set by the government. Instead, they depend on how much your body needs and how much you can absorb. If your gut microbiome is depleted, you will have a far greater nutritional requirement than what is considered normal.

Dr Abram Hoffer and Dr Andrew Saul have published many books on Orthomolecular Medicine. For many years, they have extolled the virtues of mega-vitamin therapy to treat diseases. The Orthomolecular Society has collected a large volume of published literature from scientists who have cured patients of various conditions by supplementing them with extremely high doses of nutritional supplements. Unfortunately, the orthomolecular proponents have suffered much vilification and criticism in attempts to discredit their work and findings. This may be due to the common human propensity to attack what we do not understand, even without investigating first to discover if it has a sound basis. However, it could also be because the findings have the potential to provide cheaper, safer, alternative treatments that will disrupt the status quo (and deplete the profits of certain big industries).

Before the breakthrough in understanding the microbiome, no one could explain why mega-vitamin doses worked so well. Now that we know the role of the microbiome in digesting nutrients, it is apparent that lacking certain microbes means you need a far higher dose of nutrients to absorb your requirement. This is where orthomolecular treatment levels shine. Those who have successfully used these protocols to cure people should finally start to receive the validation and recognition they deserve.

In Detoxification

Microbes also have a vital role in breaking down toxins, such as heavy metals and other contaminants, and eliminating them from the body via their bacterial pathways. If the microbes cannot break down and eliminate them, these toxins will build up, causing your liver and other organs to become congested trying to deal with the onslaught. This will often show as skin breakouts and chemical sensitivities. Many people have advocated that eczema is caused by liver congestion; this is one of the spider legs in the system, but the deeper issue is the gut dysbiosis that allows the liver congestion to develop in the first place. The reason liver cleansing regimes can (in some cases) improve eczema is because the dietary changes involved simultaneously help heal the gut and enhance the microbiome.

High levels of heavy metals in the blood are linked to the development of neurological problems in later life, have been shown to impair the production of healthy skin, and are implicated in many other disease states. When dealing with eczema, if a predisposing gene mutation is present, inflammatory cytokines further suppressing the expression of S100 skin proteins, and a gut dysbiosis that impairs your ability to absorb amino acids, the last thing needed is toxicity further interfering with your ability to produce an effective skin barrier. I talk about toxicity further and how to detox safely in Chapter 12.

In Vaccine Immune Response

Our gut microbiome directly influences our response to vaccines.

Changes in the gut microbiome can leave people at higher risk of vaccine injury or ineffective immune response. It would be far safer to test for gut dysbiosis before administering vaccines, but this is highly unlikely due to the prohibitive cost.

Scientific studies have shown that infant gut dysbiosis causes systemic inflammation and a greater likelihood of adverse vaccine effects, particularly the absence of Bifidobacterium strains. (37)

In mouse studies, five vaccines were explicitly shown to yield impaired immune responses after inducing gut dysbiosis by administering antibiotics to infant mice. These vaccines were:

- Meningococcal Serogroup B (Bexsero)
- Meningococcal Serogroup C (Neis Vac C)
- 13 valent pneumococcal conjugate vaccine (Prevenar)
- Hexavalent combination, hep B, diphtheria, tetanus, pertussis, HIB (Infanrix Hexa)
- BCG vaccine

In all cases, early exposure to antibiotics resulted in impaired antibody responses. At the same time, the production of inflammatory helper T cell cytokines was not reduced in the mice. This type of impairment in immune function causes increased inflammation without the benefit of making adequate antibodies to fight the future infections the vaccines were supposed to protect against. The impaired immune response in the mice was shown to be dependent on antibiotic-driven gut dysbiosis rather than any direct effects of the antibiotics themselves. The study stated that: "Restoration of the commensal microbiota following antibiotic exposure rescued these impaired responses." (21) This is wonderful news. If repairing the gut microbiota in mice can rescue their immune responses, correct antibody responses, and reduce inflammatory cytokines, restoring our own gut microbiota could also rescue our immune system responses.

With microbiome dysbiosis negatively affecting the ability to detoxify, this also raises serious concerns about the impact of heavy metals administered as adjuvants in the vaccines. I will discuss the effects of these in further detail in the chapter on toxicity.

In Emotional Well-being

Our gut microbes also help make many neurotransmitters, which are essential for our brain health and emotional well-being. Quite simply, having a healthy, diverse gut microbe community means you feel happier and more peaceful. However, I must re-iterate; your gut microbes cannot make the neurotransmitters for the brain if they are not there!

Gut dysbiosis reduces the production of gamma-aminobutyric acid, serotonin (the happy hormone), and other neurotransmitters, leading to depression, anxiety, and other neurological disorders. This triggers a stress response in the brain, initiating the 'fight or flight' response. The changes cause increased anxiety, fear, and insecurity responses, which are linked to increased inflammation, a suppressed innate immune response, Th2 dominance, and an increased IgE allergy response. Gut dysbiosis also leads to reductions in short-chain fatty acids; these are substances produced by our gut microbes when they digest certain complex carbohydrates. An example of a short-chain fatty acid is butyrate, which is necessary for maintaining the integrity of the gut lining. Without sufficient butyrate, the gut lining can deteriorate, leading to a leaky gut, and increased chronic inflammation in the body.

Clostridium species are the primary producers of short-chain fatty acids. The chronic stress, anxiety, and depression that many eczema patients experience can be caused by the depletion of these microbes and are not just the effects of dealing with eczema. *Lactobacilli* are poor producers of short-chain fatty acids but strong producers of lactic acid, which is rapidly converted to butyrate by other microbiota members. (21) These colonies are essential for maintaining the gut lining and preventing gut inflammation.

In Weight Management

Our gut microbiome significantly impacts our metabolism, resulting in changes to our weight and the risk of obesity. Scientists have discovered that some microbes help people to stay slim. In experiments on mice, when scientists removed certain microbes from their guts, they became obese, even though they ate the same food and did the same exercise as before. In addition, an overpopulation of pathogenic yeast microbes, such as *Candida*, can not only cause cravings for sugar, leading to weight increase but also increase systemic inflammation, which can cause weight gain.

In Immunity

In his brilliant book "The Beautiful Cure", Daniel M. Davis explains how the immune system adjusts its behaviour to maintain different bacteria levels in the gut. The cells switch on or off in response to small molecules called metabolites, which are natural biproducts of the growth and replication of gut bacteria. Think of metabolites as being like exhaust fumes from a running vehicle. Some species produce exhaust fumes recognised by your immune system as being from dirty, undesirable vehicles, and others produce exhaust fumes that are quite beneficial.

Vast numbers of helper T cells reside in your gut; they constantly monitor the metabolites released by the various microbes. The friendly microbes produce different metabolites from the unfriendly ones. Thus, these helper T cells can assess the balance of metabolites. If the pathogenic microbes in your gut are becoming too prevalent, helper T cells put your immune system on high alert, which increases systemic inflammation. When the metabolites from your commensurate or friendly microbes are within the proper ratios, the helper T cells produce anti-inflammatory molecules to calm your immune system, which reduces inflammation. It also counteracts their tendency to switch on in the presence of other less harmful bacteria elsewhere in the body. If these commensurate microbes have been depleted, they cannot produce enough metabolites to trigger the production of anti-inflammatory cytokines by your helper T cells. Therefore, they cannot dampen down your immune response, and it just keeps raging. It can even overreact when it encounters other strains of bacteria elsewhere. This is how your gut can suppress the production of inflammatory cytokines IL-6 and TNF-α, as I mentioned earlier.

Dr Davis explains, "If the metabolite levels from these favoured microbes fall, then the immune cells take this as a cue that unwanted, potentially harmful bacteria may have begun to displace the normal healthy flora. The immune system kicks into action to defend us and our resident gut bacteria." Awesome stuff! It is like you have Star Wars-type battles going on inside you every day.

In addition, gut dysbiosis has been shown to predispose infants to developing eczema. Those seen to be at the highest risk for developing atopic dermatitis by two years of age had reduced colonisation of *Bifidobacterium*, Akkermansia, *Faecalibacterium,* and *Lactobacillus*, in addition to having higher than normal populations of *Candida* and *Rhototorula* fungi. This imbalance helps to drive the inflammatory response by encouraging the differentiation of helper T cells to the more inflammatory Th2 type seen to be predominant in childhood allergic diseases. (5, 11)

In Gene Expression

The environment in your gut also influences gene expression through epigenetics. We previously believed that our genes encoded our diseases for life, and if we had a gene mutation predisposing us to certain conditions, then it was almost a given that we would develop them. We now know that disease genes can be switched off, or at the very least turned down, and other healing, regenerating genes can be switched on. However, we can only achieve this in the right microbial environment. If microbes responsible for regulating our epigenetic environment are not present or have been depleted, they are unable to provide the right conditions to flip those switches to allow you to heal.

In Hormone Production

Yes, your microbiome can help to regulate hormone levels too, and can even regulate hormone production. For example, they can replace declining estrogen production during and after menopause. Perhaps if we had not destroyed so much of the rainforest inside us and had instead nurtured our gut colonies more effectively, women would not suffer so many symptoms of menopause. Is it a coincidence that those nations where women eat a wide variety of plant foods, particularly fermented foods, do not appear to suffer from many menopausal symptoms that Western women experience? I think not.

As estrogen production from the ovaries declines, the gut microbes should produce the hormone to compensate for the reduction. That depends on whether they are there in sufficient numbers to do so. As a side note for women of childbearing age suffering from eczema, it is helpful to be aware that the cyclical drop in estrogen during your monthly cycle can cause additional moisture loss and dryness in your skin. Keep track of your cycle and be extra vigilant with your moisturising and histidine supplementation around this time.

Having a happy and diverse microbiome keeps us alive and healthy. You can see from the small list above how essential they are to our survival. But please also remember that these are not their only actions. Scientists have yet to discover all the roles our microbes perform, very much like those studying the species that reside in the Amazon Rainforest.

With these amazing organisms working inside us, we should be extremely healthy. Yet we have more chronic sickness than any generation in history. What has gone wrong?

The Seven Biggest Microbiome Killers

Just as human interference and greed have caused much destruction to the Amazon Rainforest, the same is true with our microbiomes. Mankind thought they were being wise, progressive, and productive when they began to destroy acres upon acres of forest to gain land for agricultural purposes. It is only now that we are beginning to realise that our supposed wisdom was foolishness and that our actions have far-reaching consequences. Similarly, mankind, in their supposed progression and cleverness, has instigated changes that have destroyed whole areas of our microbiome, wiping out species to the point of extinction and causing untold destruction to the 'rainforest' within.

Allow me to expose the seven biggest microbiome killers. As you read these, you will identify many of them in your own life and start to recognise how your gut dysbiosis has likely occurred.

1. Antibiotics

The first big killer of our microbiome is antibiotics. Antibiotics were a great discovery and have saved countless lives, but they have unfortunately been over-prescribed and over-used. They have also been prescribed in situations for which they are ineffective, such as viral infections. This misuse has not only created antibiotic-resistant diseases as pathogens adapt to survive the antibiotic culture, but it has also depleted our microbiomes to the point that it is now affecting our offspring. Mothers can only pass on the microbes they have themselves.

The word antibiotic is derived from a compound of two words, 'anti' meaning against, and 'biotic' meaning life. So, antibiotic literally translates to 'against life'. The idea of antibiotics is to kill the pathogenic bacterium causing sickness. However, antibiotics are indiscriminate killers, and the friendly bacterium of the microbiome are the innocent casualties during their use. A single dose of antibiotic medication can wipe out whole colonies. Unfortunately for us, these commensurate organisms typically take far longer to recover than any pathogenic ones; gut dysbiosis is often the result. Gut dysbiosis simply means that your gut microbes are out of balance with the proliferation of pathogenic ones compared to commensurate ones. Dysbiosis results in numerous health issues. The risk of dysbiosis is even more significant in the guts of infants whose microflora is still developing and establishing itself. Even if you think you are doing well because you have not had a course of antibiotics for a while, you are most likely consuming antibiotics every single day without even being aware of it. Yes, there are hidden antibiotics everywhere.

Consider preservatives in packaged food. What are they designed to do? Preserve food. How do they do this? By killing the bacteria that would cause the food to spoil. Therefore, preservatives function as antibiotics, with the same detrimental side effects on your microbiome when you eat them. However, because they are called preservatives on the list of ingredients rather than antibiotics, most people are entirely unaware that they are consuming microbe-harming antibiotics.

Another source of hidden antibiotics is conventionally farmed meat. Industrial farming methods involve keeping the animals cramped in indoor stalls and cages, feeding them unnatural diets, such as genetically modified soya, and depriving them of sunlight. This enforced unhealthy lifestyle causes the animals to be chronically sick. Cows, for example, are genetically hardwired to be outside in the sunshine, eating chlorophyll-rich grasses full of antioxidants and micro-RNAs. Healthy animals in their natural environment are not riddled with disease and chronic inflammation like factory-farmed animals tend to be. Antibiotics are commonly used as prophylactic medications to keep intensively farmed animals from developing the inevitable bacterial infections that result from their enforced unhealthy lifestyle and to treat the mastitis that typically develops in sick milk cows. We then eat these animals or consume their milk or eggs, like chickens, and as a result, we also consume the antibiotic residues in them.

Pasteurisation and heat-treatment protocols are forms of antibiotic treatments designed to kill bacteria in foods. They may not kill the bacteria directly in the gut. However, they kill the food's commensurate beneficial bacteria while destroying the pathogenic ones, thereby preventing us from replenishing the friendly microbe colonies in our guts.

The view of all bacteria being pathogenic has created a fear of microbes and the need to zealously eradicate them with all types of antibacterial cleaning agents and antibiotics. We seek to eliminate them from our homes with toxic cleaning agents; from our food with preservatives, irradiation, and pasteurisation; and from our bodies with antibacterial cleansing agents and sanitisers. We prevent our kids from playing where they will become inculcated with more beneficial microbes because we do not want them getting dirty, even though the beneficial microbes that guard our health originated in that environment, such as unadulterated soil and air. In doing our best to protect ourselves and our families from unwanted and unseen bacterial 'threats', we are inadvertently creating dysbiosis in our bodies and those of our children.

Whether they are used to clean surfaces, hands, or laundry, antibacterial sanitisers are also antibiotics. We have demonised bacteria to the extent that we view every bacterium as a threat to be annihilated, whereas many of them actually help to keep us healthy. When we sterilise our environment, we rob ourselves of the opportunity to replenish the good microbes. Hand sanitisers are a problem now that everyone is forced to sanitise multiple times daily. As we learnt in 'The Riddle of The Root', healthy skin produces its own antibacterial protection, but hand sanitisers destroy these microbes while killing pathogens. There are many ways to utilise natural cleaning agents to keep our homes and bodies clean without stripping them of all bacterial life forms. The Environmental Working Group website (ewg.org) is a great tool to help you source non-toxic products of all types.

Chlorine in water is yet another hidden antibiotic which kills microbes indiscriminately. When we bathe in and drink chlorinated water, we destroy the commensurate microbes on our skin and in our guts. The pathogens recover faster, and then the skin is left with higher-than-normal levels of *Staphylococcus,* eliciting such a strong immune response that it can cause an eczema rash on previously healthy skin. Our gut microbe communities are also detrimentally affected by drinking chlorinated water; this explains why those who regularly consume chlorinated water have a significantly increased cancer risk, as detailed in the study published by The Food Revolution Network that I mentioned earlier in the book.

There are microbiome-friendly, natural antibiotics we can utilise to treat infections, such as my family's go-to: raw garlic, which kills pathogenic bacteria whilst simultaneously feeding gut microbes as a prebiotic rather than harming them. Again, I suggest doing your research. There are alternatives available to you that are safer than pharmaceutical medications. Consulting with a natural health professional will help you discover what options are available to you for your circumstances.

If we want to preserve our precious microbiome and well-being, we cannot afford to remain ignorant of what we put on and in our bodies. Nor can we live in a sterile environment if we wish to be healthy.

2. C-sections and Bottle-feeding

If you visit a doctor who practices a more holistic model of medicine, for example, integrative or functional medicine, you may be surprised how far their interest in antibiotic exposure and the microbiome goes back. It is not uncommon for them to ask whether you were born by C-section or vaginal birth; if your mother was given intravenous or prophylactic antibiotics before giving birth or when she was breast feeding; whether your mother breastfed you at all; or whether you (or your child) were given antibiotics before the age of 3 years old. All these will affect the microbiome, even into adulthood. A mother can only pass on what she has within herself. If her own 'rainforest' has been decimated, there will be 'tribes and species' that the new infant will not inherit.

C-sections have saved countless babies and mothers in emergencies; however, babies born by C-sections are known to have a much lower level of innate immunity and are at higher risk of infections, especially respiratory and atopic diseases. This is directly due to the lack of microbiome populating infants as they emerge into the world. Awareness of this problem is growing; thankfully, some maternity units now take swabs from the mother's birth canal and wipe the fluid all over the C-section babies to cover them in the necessary microbes. This is an effective protocol to improve the immune function of these infants.

Another common problem in the maternity wards is the frequent use of prophylactic antibiotics in longer labours *just in case* an infection arises that could put the baby at risk. This practice destroys the colonies of bacteria that the mother's body prepared for the infant to pick up on their way out, leaving the children at higher risk of respiratory disease and atopic disease in a similar way to if they had been born by C-section. Obviously, there are cases when antibiotics must be administered, for example, if the mother tests possible for *Streptococcus B* infection, but prophylactic antibiotics should not be indiscriminately used without first testing to see if an infection actually does exist. It may appear to be an effective and cheap preventative protocol. Still, it leads to long-term detrimental depletion of both the numbers and diversity of microbes colonising the infants. This, in turn, is creating untold numbers of children with lower immunity and at higher risk of health issues. There are multitudes of scientific documents revealing the effects of infant gut dysbiosis on everything, including disease risk, future obesity, atopic risk, and altered vaccine response. This practice seriously needs to be reconsidered. If it does prove necessary to administer antibiotics to a pregnant or labouring woman, then probiotics should also be administered to restore the gut microflora in both the mother and the child.

A study conducted in 2016 indicated that the infant group at the highest risk of developing issues such as asthma, eczema, and allergic responses have a gut microbiome that promotes adaptive immune dysfunction associated with atopy. The study suggested that manipulating the infant's gut microbiota with probiotic supplements directly influences the child's susceptibility to develop childhood atopy, particularly allergies and asthma. Furthermore, interventions to alter the gut microbiome environment showed positive impacts on the ability of the helper T cells to change the composition and function of the gut microbiome. The conclusion was that probiotic intervention may offer a viable strategy for disease prevention in babies and children. (11) Although the researchers published this excellent study in 2016, eczema patients and those with atopic conditions are still not being told that this treatment option even exists. It certainly is not being utilised in maternity units and pediatric clinics.

When scientists analysed the gut microbes in infants, they found that the early gut colonisers of healthy babies typically include commensal facultative anaerobes such as *Enterobacter* and *Enterococci*. (Facultative anaerobes are microbes that produce energy in the form of adenosine triphosphate, otherwise known as ATP, by respiration when oxygen is present in their environment, but can also switch to producing energy by fermentation when no oxygen is present.) These microbes are followed by an increased relative abundance of strict anaerobes (oxygen respirating microbes), including *Bifidobacterium, Bacteroides,* and *Clostridium.* The gut microbiota is dominated by the *Firmicutes* and *Bacteroidetes* bacterial strains and, to a lesser extent, *Proteobacteria, Actinobacteria,* and *Verrucomicrobia.* These, along with *Bifidobacterium, Lactobacillus, Faecalibacterium,* and *Akkermansia,* are the strains that pediatric doctors should be prescribing to manipulate the guts of infants and children to reduce their risk of developing atopic conditions.

Bacterial colonies usually reside in different areas along the gastrointestinal tract as their location is strongly influenced by the nutrient distribution of their preferred food source. For example, *Proteobacteria* and *Lactobacillus* are present in the small intestine because monosaccharides, disaccharides, and amino acids, which represent their primary food source, are present in this sector. Beyond the ileocecal valve, which separates your small and large intestines, the community changes because most of the carbohydrates available are polysaccharides that *Proteobacteria* cannot digest and use as energy. In contrast, *Bacteroides* and *Clostridial* have enzymes that can break down these undigested polysaccharides and digest them by fermentation. These fermentation processes produce acetate, propionate (*Bacteroides*), and butyrate (*Firmicutes*), which play essential roles in maintaining a healthy gut. (21)

Scientists have found that the highest risk group for the development of eczema by two years of age showed reduced colonisation of *Bifidobacterium, Akkermansia, Faecalibacterium,* and *Lactobacillus,* plus an excess of *Candida* and *Rhototorula* fungi, creating a distinct faecal metabolome perfect for producing high pro-inflammatory metabolites. A microbial dysbiosis of this sort drives the helper T cells to differentiate into the more inflammatory Th2 type, which is associated with the development of childhood atopy, particularly when the gut displays deficient levels of *Bifidobacterium, Lactobacillus, Faecalibacterium,* and *Akkermansia.* (11)

The lowest risk group had more abundant polyunsaturated fatty acids, succinate, and important components of breast milk called oligosaccharides (3-fucosyllactose and lacto-N-focupentaose: specific forms of carbohydrate found in breast milk). These are known to influence the health of the gut epithelial lining. (11)

Breast milk contains the sugars mentioned above, oligosaccharides and lactose, in addition to over 1,000 indigestible molecules. These were previously thought to be useless compounds; however, we now know that they provide food sources for the microbial communities in the infant's gut, allowing their communities to be established and flourish. These communities digest those molecules through their fermentation processes and release beneficial compounds into the infant's body for their health and development. For example, galactooligosaccharides act as growth stimulators for *Bifidobacterium* and improve the intestinal environment making it more conducive for them to thrive. (20) These compounds continue to benefit us throughout our lives, not just as infants. Hence, scientists recommend exclusive breastfeeding for a minimum of 4 months (16). This helps to create a less inflammatory microbiome terrain in the infant's gut and reduces the risk of developing atopic diseases.

The microbiome is particularly unstable during the first three years of life as several factors highly modulate it. It can also be impacted throughout the rest of life, although any damage caused in the early years has far more significant consequences. The first two years of life are defined as the critical window where the instability of microbiota is likely to reflect in the plasticity of the immune system. The third year is also considered equally important by some researchers. Microbial imbalance can predispose the body to disease, including *Clostridium difficile* infections, metabolic and neuropsychiatric disorders, rheumatoid diseases, and microbiota dysbiosis-related diseases in other areas of the body, such as cystic fibrosis, chronic rhinosinusitis, periodontal issues, and pain and central nervous system disorders. (21) Studies have shown that infants with insufficient colonisation of beneficial microbes are at increased risk of developing auto-immune diseases, not just atopic diseases such as allergies, asthma, eczema, and allergic rhinitis, but also late-onset sepsis and coronary heart disease. (37)

Putting newly born infants first onto hospital scales for weighing and measuring and then to the hospital crib is also not beneficial for their microbiome. Unless there are medical reasons why hospital staff need to remove infants from their mothers immediately after birth, infants should first be given direct skin-to-skin contact with their mothers to help populate healthy colonies of microbes on their skin. If the infant is first placed on hospital scales or cribs, it is highly likely the infant's skin will populate with *Staphylococcus* and other pathogenic microbes during its first contact with the world. This practice also dramatically increases their risk of developing eczema, particularly if they have not inherited a diverse microbiome during birth.

If born by C-section or exposed to antibiotics during labour, there is a much greater risk of developing eczema and allergies. If, for whatever reason, breastfeeding did not occur, this risk compounds further. (11) I am not condemning anyone for the choices they have either made or been forced into concerning labour or infant feeding. My purpose here is not to judge but to help you identify the risk factors and roots for your own or your child's development of eczema. We cannot change the past, but by gaining knowledge, we can take action to mitigate the risk factors or correct any damage. In a similar way to when we are lost, we must first discover where we are before we can plan how to get to where we want to be. By helping you find out where you are, I can help direct you to the right paths to get you back on track with your health.

3. Non-Steroidal Anti-Inflammatory Drug Painkillers

Non-steroidal anti-inflammatory drugs include ibuprofen and aspirin. They are frequently taken for pain and fever relief and are often available without prescription as over-the-counter medicines in pharmacies. In September 2014, Dawn Connelly published an interesting article on the website of Pharmaceutical-journal.com titled: "A History of Aspirin". According to Connelly, aspirin was developed after researchers sought to discover why ancient civilisations used willow bark to relieve their aches and pains. As far back as 3000 B.C., ancient papyrus records show Sumerians and Egyptians using willow as their go-to anti-inflammatory. Hippocrates used willow-leaf tea to ease the pains of women in labour at around 400 B.C. However, it was not until 1828 that the active ingredient responsible for its pain-relieving qualities was isolated, named salicin. Two years later, researchers discovered salicin in meadow sweet flowers. In 1853, a French chemist, Charles Frederic Gerhardt, determined salicylic acid's chemical (molecular) structure and created a synthetic copy called acetylsalicylic acid, which was then patented in 1899 and marketed as aspirin. As interesting as the article is, it falls short of addressing any of the side effects of aspirin and instead focuses on its history and virtues. In clinical trials, aspirin has been shown to cause damage to the stomach and intestinal lining, leading to the development of erosions, ulcers, and stomach perforations. (36)

Following research during the 1950s and 1960s to find a supposedly safer alternative to aspirin, ibuprofen was developed. However, ibuprofen is also known to cause damage to the gastrointestinal tract and to increase the risk of heart failure, kidney failure, and liver failure. It has also been shown to worsen asthma, so its reputation as being safer than aspirin is highly questionable. Here lies the difficulty of trying to manufacture isolated compounds from nature to sell as medicine.

Those who used willow bark in the ancient civilisations did not suffer the gastrointestinal issues that come from using aspirin today. This is because willow bark, in its whole state, contains other substances that protect the gut lining. It would be fantastic if, when scientists discover beneficial medicinal compounds in a plant, the authorities invested resources into growing an abundance of those plants for the benefit of humanity. However, as natural plants cannot be patented and sold for huge profits, this will not occur. Instead, we will continue to isolate only the effective compound. Unfortunately, this produces inferior treatments that commonly lack the other naturally protective compounds that exist in nature. However, these treatments can be patented and sold as pharmaceutical drugs for high profits. Unfortunately, those who take them continue to suffer the side effects of using them. How sad that we have so many beautiful remedies in nature, but modern medicine has branded herbalism and natural medicine as quackery to discredit it and instead trumpets only pharmaceutical remedies as acceptable mainstream medicine. In the meantime, the general population pops pain-killing medication like candy and then suffers the consequences of using it. These painkillers will damage your gastrointestinal tract and cause detrimental changes to the gut microflora. If you are interested in discovering real, natural painkillers, I highly recommend subscribing to or joining Green Med Info (www. greenmedinfo.com), the brainchild of Sayer Ji, who has collated many thousands of science documents detailing proven natural protocols for treating pain and disease.

An excellent natural, anti-inflammatory supplement is available online. Although it is not cheap, it is both natural and highly effective. I used it myself when we first moved to Trinidad on missionary service. The mosquitos seemed particularly attracted to me, and unfortunately, I suffered from severe reactions to the mosquito bites; every bite would swell to the size of a side plate. I was in torment! Nothing I tried worked to relieve the itching, swelling, and pain until I found a supplement online called Bosmeric. It is the invention of Sunil Pai, MD and comprises frankincense, ginger, curcumin, and a black pepper extract called peperine. Not only did it work effectively when nothing else had, but it also did so very quickly, bringing down the swelling, reducing the pain, and stopping the itching, all without any nasty side effects. I also used Bosmeric for pain relief after recent dental surgery involving both a tooth extraction and a crown. The dentist was so impressed by my pain management he took a photograph of the Bosmeric pot to share with his other holistic patients. I am not affiliated with Sunil Pai or his products; I am simply sharing this experience with you to show you there are effective anti-inflammatories available that do not cause damage to your health.

4. Pesticides

Glyphosate (Roundup™) and pesticides used in non-organic agricultural farming are also a form of antibiotics. You cannot simply rinse the pesticides off your fruit and vegetables as the chemicals run into the ground and are then absorbed into the stems of the plants as they uptake the water and nutrients from the soil. Then they are IN the plants, not just ON the plants. The pesticides were initially marketed as safe for human consumption as they did not show detrimental effects on human cells in lab tests. However, the bacterial pathways targeted by these pesticides to kill insects are the same ones used by the gut's commensurate (friendly) bacteria. Therefore, by eating pesticide-laden foods, we are contributing to the destruction of our 'internal rainforest' and many native species with critical roles in maintaining our health. Unfortunately, pesticides and herbicides are hidden ingredients in many of our foods; there is no requirement to list them, so until someone points them out to us, we remain largely unaware of their existence. Organic food is far safer, and the most effective way to force change in our agricultural practices is to wield the power of our wallets. Quite simply, what we refuse to buy will no longer be profitable to produce. Remember that in business, profits determine decisions. Where you spend your money affects what is profitable to make and what is not. Recently, I was dismayed to learn that less than 3% of the agricultural land in the United Kingdom is farmed organically. We can change this. The more people buy organic produce, the more we create demand for it, and the more viable it becomes for farmers to convert their land to organic. This not only gives us more choices of organic food but also reduces the environmental damage from all the agricultural chemicals polluting our air, food, and waterways.

5. The Westernized Diet

The 'Standard American Diet' is nicknamed the 'SAD' diet, not just because it is an anagram of the letters, but because it literally does make people sad. This way of eating starves the microbiome through nutritionally dead food and has largely contributed to the epidemic of anxiety, depression, and mental illness by depleting our microbes and detrimentally affecting their ability to produce neurotransmitters, such as serotonin. These neurotransmitters are vital for various functions, such as regulating our mood, anxiety levels, sleep patterns, and appetite, to name a few. I previously stated that our microbes live in a symbiotic relationship with us, meaning we are supposed to look after them too. We need to eat foods that feed them, namely fresh organic plants and good quality proteins. Our gut microbiomes

DO NOT like sugar, fried foods, processed food, refined carbohydrates, and too much meat. The typical high-sugar, highly processed Western diet starves our microbes of the nutrients they need and, at the same time, starves us of the beneficial compounds they would produce if they were digesting their preferred foods. Eating lots of organic plants helps create the ideal environment for the health-promoting microbes to thrive inside us, which are also valuable sources of both probiotics and prebiotics. (Prebiotics are the food sources for the probiotics). I remember whenever I was pregnant, I would constantly check how the foods I ate would affect my baby. Well, we need to all eat like we are pregnant and be mindful of how our choices affect the microbes in our gut. But instead of eating for two, we are eating for trillions.

The Western diet has abandoned traditional food preparation and storage methods, which also impacts the health of our microbiome. In times past, we would preserve our food using cultural methods handed down through generations of wisdom, like fermenting and curing in salt. Countries that still eat ancestral diets typically ferment their foods to preserve them, like kimchi in Korea and natto in Japan. These fermented foods are teeming with probiotics that, when eaten regularly, help to keep the commensurate bacteria colonies at healthy levels. Think of fermented foods as being like the Sahara dust that regularly blows across the ocean to replenish and fertilise the soil of the Amazon. In contrast to traditional preservation methods, modern storage methods involve sterilising, pasteurising, heat treating, irradiation techniques, and using chemical preservatives in everything packaged. The old ways encouraged the growth of beneficial microbes in the food, which enabled us to replenish our gut microbes every time we ate. Nowadays, we eat food that is not only devoid of any significant probiotic benefit but which is also loaded with artificial additives to compound the problem. For example, artificial sweeteners and additives such as sucralose, aspartame, carrageenan, polysorbate 80, titanium dioxide, maltodextrin, and sodium sulphites have all been shown to disturb the balance of our gut microbes. (74)

6. Stress

We currently live in a stressful world, not only because of continued Covid-19 restrictions but also due to the perceived threats that create a constant state of high alert in our stress response system: financial insecurities, concerns about the health of loved ones or ourselves, fears of being the victim of a crime or getting caught in a terrorist attack, stressful work environments, family breakdowns, the list is never-ending. Chronic stress disturbs the gut environment as it switches on your body's 'fight or flight' mechanism, shutting down processes that are not immediately important. This allows you to divert that energy to stay alive. If you are under threat, the digestive and healing systems are not the most important things. Therefore, to conserve your energy to either fight or run, other less urgent functions get put on hold until the threat has passed. If your digestion is being shut down regularly by chronic stress, this will affect the health of your gut colonies. I have devoted an entire chapter to how stress impacts eczema, where we will examine this in more detail.

7. Lack of Exercise

Exercise has numerous proven benefits, including increased oxygen intake because of faster breathing, which benefits your whole body, including all your cells. Another advantage of intentional movement is that it causes your lymph fluid to move through your lymph system faster. This speeds up the process of waste removal, which helps keep us healthy and assists in preventing excess histamine release caused by constipation. On the other hand, sedentary lives can lead to inefficiency in toxin removal, and the build-up of toxins can adversely affect our microbiome.

What Can We Do?

Clearly, we need to protect our microbiomes, but we cannot escape modern life. So, what can we do? Now that you know what the biggest killers of your microbiome are, you can take measures to minimise your exposure to them. Buy organic produce as much as possible.

Try to avoid unnecessary antibiotic exposure. Reduce dependency on non-steroidal anti-inflammatory medications and seek a holistic medical practitioner for alternative pain relief. Start making efforts to transition back to a natural diet, free from processed and artificial foods. Buying foods and ingredients still in their natural, unadulterated form will go a long way in protecting your health. Check online for easy at-home fermenting recipes, and start making your own Lacto-fermented veggies to replenish your microbiome. Remember to ensure home-fermented foods are kept underneath the brine to prevent histamine production, as previously explained. In addition, start getting active with intentional exercise. We will look at stress-relieving strategies in Chapter 11, as stress has its own loop systems to address and unravel.

Do Probiotic Supplements Help?

Will taking probiotics help to heal eczema? Yes, it will, and its benefits are not restricted to eczema alone. Restoring the correct gut microflora in your gut will positively impact your immune system, brain, emotions, hormones, and many other areas. Rather than give my opinion though, let me share a sample of the evidence published in scientific papers.

One study examined the rates of eczema in countries around the world. Interestingly, they found the lowest rates of eczema across all age groups in Japan. (19) I am sure it is no coincidence that Japan has one of the highest probiotic diets in the world, with the consumption of natto, miso, and tofu, as well as one of the lowest number of required vaccinations for infants.

Another study published in 2012 assessed the effects of probiotics given to pregnant and breastfeeding mothers in families known to be at high risk of developing atopic diseases. They concluded that supplementing with probiotics does reduce the risk of infants developing eczema and atopy, stating that: "Early intervention to manipulate gut microbiota may offer a viable strategy for disease prevention. Studies show a reduced risk of atopy by supplementing *Lactobacillus rhamnosus*

(HN001) and *Bifidobacterium animalis* (subspecies lactis HN019). Probiotic mixtures with different strains of bacteria were seen to be superior in their effects to monotherapy (meaning the supplements with many different strains were more effective than those using just one single strain)." (13)

A study in 2003 found that probiotic treatment was shown to skew the helper T cell balance by inhibiting the production of Th2 cytokines. (12) Remember that Th2 cytokines are heavily involved in the inflammatory cycle of eczema. The article went on to state that there are multiple mechanisms by which probiotics decrease atopic tendencies, not just the skewing of Th1/Th2 balance towards Th1 by inhibiting the Th2 inflammatory cytokines, but also by directly increasing anti-inflammatory IL-10 cytokines and regulatory T cell (Treg) production through either dendritic cell maturation or toll-like receptors. (12)

The same researchers stated that the probiotic strain *Lactobacillus rhamnosus* has been used successfully to reduce peanut allergy and cow's milk allergies in children. The effect was most significant if it was given before the infants were six months of age. (12)

Lactobacillus rhamnosus was also the subject of another study published in 2014 titled "Effects of *Lactobacillus Rhamnosus* on Allergic March." They found that people who showed high levels of inflammatory cytokines and thymic stromal lymphopoietin showed immune responses associated with the progression of the Allergic March. However, these responses were suppressed by treatment with *Lactobacillus Rhamnosus (Lcr35)*. Moreover, when mice who showed Allergic March phenotypes were treated with *Lactobacillus Rhamnosus (Lcr35)*, they showed an increase in the number of anti-inflammatory helper T cells and Tregs in their lymph nodes. In conclusion, the authors of the study stated that oral supplementation of *Lactobacillus Rhamnosus (Lcr35)* prevented the development of the Allergic March by suppressing Th2 differentiation, inflammatory cytokine production, and thymic stromal lymphopoietin. (34) Bearing in mind this was published in 2014 and was very effective, you would think this would have been communicated to every medic treating atopic patients. I can only assume that it was not because it was not profitable enough to do so. I cannot think of any other viable explanation. It is far more lucrative to develop various immunosuppressant drugs.

One excellent study, published in April 2016, states that "the application of probiotics reduced inflammation by suppressing the production of both IL-4 inflammatory cytokines, and the differentiation of inflammatory helper T cell types, and increasing the expression of IL-10 and Treg-related anti-inflammatory cytokines. Probiotics also inhibit the maturing of the naïve dendritic cells (when they 'wake- up' in the presence of thymic stromal lymphopoietin and migrate to the lymph system to recruit more inflammatory re-enforcements), which consequently inhibits the naive helper T cells from differentiating into Th2 cells. This reduces the inflammatory process in the skin" (this is the process we covered in Chapter 7). It confirms that the differentiation of naïve helper T cells caused by the dendritic cells regulated by thymic stromal lymphopoietin causes this inflammatory cycle. The process can be inhibited, and the allergic disease can be suppressed by supplementing with probiotics. (43) All this without the need for, or side effects of, pharmaceutical medications. Now that is amazing!

In another study, published in 2010, titled *"Lactobacillus Rhamnosus Cell Lysate in the Management of Resistant Childhood Atopic Eczema"*, researchers followed 14 pediatric patients (ages eight months to 64 months) with a history of resistant eczema for at least six months. All children received 300 mg to 500 mg standardised *Lactobacillus Rhamnosus* probiotic as an immunobiotic supplement daily. The scientists stated: "The results of this open-label non-randomised clinical observation showed a substantial improvement in quality of life, skin symptoms, and day- and night-time irritation scores in children with the supplementation of *Lactobacillus rhamnosus* lysate. There were no cases of intolerance or adverse reactions observed in these children. *Lactobacillus rhamnosus* cell lysate may be used as a safe and effective immunobiotic for treating and preventing childhood eczema and possibly other types of atopy (allergic diseases)." (47) What an outstanding result that hardly anyone has heard of.

Studies have also found that supplementing the diets of mice and rats with *Lactobacillus* and *Bifidobacterium* increases gamma-aminobutyric acid production. This resulted in a decrease in depressive behaviour, a reduction of corticosterone-induced stress and anxiety, and reduced visceral pain. (45) Although this study did not mention eczema directly, stress has a considerable impact on the inflammatory state, which I will cover in Chapter 11. In addition, eczema sufferers typically show far higher stress responses and anxiety levels than normal, so the fact that probiotic supplementation can reduce anxiety and stress will mean that it will have a consequential impact on the resulting inflammation that their stress would have caused.

Finally, another study showed that pathogenic bacterial overload in the gut has been shown to increase histamine levels in the body, as the food is not broken down as quickly as it should be, causing it to produce more histamine than it should. (53) Correcting the balance of microbes will reduce the histamine burden in the gut.

In the conclusion of our discussion of probiotics, I suggest that you **should** supplement with probiotics and the earlier you do so, the better. If you are an adult suffering from eczema, it is still an effective treatment, as I mentioned earlier in the book. Probiotics have been shown to be as effective as mid-potency corticosteroids with no side effects, particularly when applied both topically to the skin and as an oral supplementation. If you are considering pregnancy, or if you are already pregnant, I would recommend supplementing with probiotics to reduce the risk of your infant developing any atopic conditions, especially if you have eczema and atopic conditions in the family.

Children and infants can safely be given probiotics. The best study results all involved the *Lactobacillus rhamnosus* strain of bacterium; however, do not look for this strain in isolation, as the studies concluded that probiotics containing a variety of species were more effective than monocultures (single strains). *Bifidobacterium animalis* was stated to be beneficial too. There are many varied strains of *Lactobacillus* and *Bifidobacterium* available that you can take safely. None of these studies found adverse side effects when supplementing with probiotics, but if you would like to seek the guidance of a medical professional, please either share this information with your doctor or look for a functional or integrative doctor who is competent in their understanding of probiotics. Show them this chapter (or even better, buy them a copy of this book so they can learn to help other eczema patients more effectively), and ask them to work with you on probiotic therapy. But please remember to implement the other legs of the eczema spider we identify in this book too.

Additional Considerations

Although our internal rainforest plays a huge role in regulating our health, healing the gut involves much more than correcting our microbiome. Many other issues can be involved, and it is important to assess the entire gut function when working to restore health. Let's look at how digestion should work and some of the common ailments that can impact the health and function of the digestive tract and consequently impact eczema.

Digestion actually starts with our eyes, not our mouths. When we prepare food, the aroma, the sight of the food, and the anticipation of eating it will signal our brain to begin producing more saliva and enzymes. (Have you noticed when you smell something sour, your mouth can start to water?) As we chew our food, we trigger the release of saliva. Saliva contains enzymes that begin to break down the starches and fats as they are mixed with the food by the process of chewing. However, not everyone chews their food effectively or produces enough saliva. This could be caused by neurological degeneration, as the chewing motion is supposed to signal the brain to trigger the release of saliva from the salivary glands. If something is amiss in the communication channels from the brain to the mouth, either by previous trauma, illness, or degeneration of the nerves or brain function, this process will be inefficient. Chewing our food sufficiently to break it up and mix it with the enzymes is an essential step in helping release the nutrients from the food for us to absorb. If you frequently feel like you have a dry mouth and need to drink lots of fluid to help you swallow your food, this could signal reduced capacity to produce saliva. Dentists sometimes identify a lack of saliva during routine check-ups, as having a dry mouth can increase the incidents of cavities and poor gum health.

Swallowing is another process involving the brain and cranial nerves and is also impacted by brain or nerve function degeneration. Anyone who develops swallowing difficulties should seek medical attention to assess for nervous system degeneration and work with a specialist who can assist them. However, most people do not have degenerative disorders. They just do not bother to chew their food properly and hurriedly swallow large chunks of food with insufficient saliva before rushing off to the next urgent task. You will help your digestion greatly by taking time to eat mindfully and chew each mouthful 10-20 times before swallowing.

The next stop on the way down the gastrointestinal tract is the stomach, which should contain enough hydrochloric acid to dissolve the food and sterilise it of pathogenic bacteria before it passes further down, where pancreatic enzymes continue the breakdown of proteins and fats. The action of chewing tells the stomach that food is on its way down and triggers the production of stomach acid and enzymes, which is another reason you need to chew your food properly. If you have low stomach acid, you will neither be able to dissolve your food effectively nor sterilise it. Bearing in mind the human body is the perfect temperature for food to spoil, if the process falls short here, your meal will start to rot inside your gut.

I talk to many people who suffer from acid reflux and are constantly burping up acidic, partially digested food. Pharmacists and their medics frequently tell them they have too much acid and should take antacids to correct the problem. As sufficient gastric acid is so vitally important for the health of the whole gastrointestinal tract, it is totally irresponsible to tell people to take antacids without first checking if they really do have excess acidity. In my experience, the problem is usually the complete opposite; they suffer from low stomach acid. Consequently, their food is fermenting inside their gut, and they are burping up gas and small amounts of partially digested food. Taking antacids only compounds the problem by reducing the stomach acid even further, whereas taking some digestive enzymes and drinking diluted apple cider vinegar or lemon juice with meals to increase the stomach acidity will often resolve the problem. I also recommend seeking professional advice about the option of taking additional hydrochloric acid as a supplement with meals if this is an issue for you.

Low stomach acid is frequently caused by chronic stress suppressing digestive functions, which I will discuss in more detail in the next chapter. However, as we consciously work to resolve the issues causing us stress or learn how to switch our stress response off, we can recover effective acid and enzyme production again. Additionally, eczema sufferers are commonly deficient in histidine. As histidine is also involved in the production of gastric acid, it is not uncommon for eczema sufferers to experience low levels of stomach acid. In this case, taking histidine supplements should help correct this and improve the skin's barrier function also.

Hypochlorhydria (low stomach acid) can also indicate other health issues, such as an underactive thyroid function, *Helicobacter pylori* infection or an undiagnosed IgG antibody reaction to Casein milk protein which can lead to a cross-reactivity or molecular mimicry immune reaction to the parietal cells of the stomach lining. All of these are relatively easy to test for. Therefore, if the symptoms I just described for low stomach acid relate to you, consider requesting these tests. Just for your information, the most accurate tests for Helicobacter pylori are either breath or stool tests. Blood tests do not accurately determine a current infection because the antibodies can remain elevated in the blood for a couple of years after a *Helicobacter pylorus* infection has been resolved. Therefore, you could be prescribed unnecessary treatment if the diagnosis is based on a blood test alone.

People with chronic inflammatory conditions, such as eczema, can also become deficient in pancreatic enzymes because these enzymes are also used elsewhere in the body to dampen inflammation. When inflammation is chronic, the pancreas may not be able to produce adequate amounts of enzymes to fight inflammation and digest food simultaneously. Regardless of the cause of low acid and enzyme production, you may need some extra support from enzyme supplements and either lemon juice, diluted apple cider vinegar, or hydrochloric acid supplements while you seek to resolve this.

The next stop on the journey down brings us to the gall bladder and the liver. The liver makes bile from cholesterol. Bile is used to break down fats. The bile is stored in the gallbladder. As the food passes down, the gallbladder contracts (another process involving the cranial nerves) to release the bile. The expelled bile also contains toxins that have been processed by the liver. The gallbladder passes these out in the bile, where they will be mixed with the waste in the bowel to pass out of the body. If the gallbladder does not contract properly to release the bile, not only will the toxins build up in the body, adversely affecting our health, but the bile in the gallbladder will also become thick and sludgy, which can then turn into gallstones. Insufficient bile will also leave us unable to digest fatty acids and fat-soluble vitamins such as A, D, E, and K. Although I have not seen any documents linking vitamin K deficiency to eczema, there are many published articles proving positive associations between deficiencies of vitamins A, D, E, and essential fatty acids, and the exhibition of eczema. A common sign of inability to digest fats is passing poop that floats. Admittedly, it is not pleasant to check one's poop, but it is advisable to look occasionally. It is surprising what you can learn about your gut health from the state of your poop.

One of the best ways to increase gallbladder activity is to increase your activity, as being sedentary or overweight is a significant risk factor for developing gallbladder dysfunction and gallstones. Eating an unhealthy high-fat, low-fibre diet or having poorly managed diabetes also contribute to impaired gallbladder function. Certain medications, such as frequent antibiotics, hormone therapy, statins, and diuretics, have also been implicated in gallstone formation.

Changing your diet to be more healthful for your microbiome, as discussed above, will also help lower your risk of developing metabolic disease and the consequent gallbladder dysfunction. Drinking coffee regularly has also been shown to be helpful as coffee helps to thin bile sludge and encourage contraction. If you are highly stressed or sensitive to caffeine, you may prefer to drink decaffeinated coffee instead. TUDCA supplements are also extremely helpful in increasing bile production to increase gut motility. Thus, they are another valuable supplement to consider.

As we continue downward, we come to the small intestine, although it is far from small, considering that it is roughly 20 feet long (6-7 meters). This part of the gastrointestinal tract is usually lined with minute finger-like structures called microvilli. If you could unzip your intestines and lay them out flat, they would look rather like a long shaggy carpet. In healthy individuals, the shags are packed tightly together to prevent undigested food particles and bacteria from leaking out of the gut into the surrounding tissues. Our blood vessels come right up to the lining of our intestines, so anything leaking out can quickly enter the bloodstream. As our blood is pumped all around our body, any leaked particles will also travel around and soon encounter immune cells in our lymph nodes, triggering an undesirable immune response. In my previous book, ' Superheroes Inside Me ', I show the effects of a leaky gut in an easy-to-understand story form. The enzyme I mentioned earlier in Chapter 8, diamine oxidase, also plays a role in hindering histamine from passing through the lining of the gut into the bloodstream. Deficiencies in this enzyme will allow higher histamine levels to enter the blood and contribute to the conditions leading to histamine intolerance, as we discussed earlier.

When the small intestine's lining is inflamed, spaces develop between the microvilli and the epithelial lining cells, allowing leakages to occur. Many substances commonly cause inflammation in the lining of the small intestine. Highly processed foods packed full of preservatives and artificial additives, gluten, excess sugar, and alcohol consumption are all known triggers, as are antibiotics, antacids, and corticosteroids. *Helicobacter pylori* infection; overpopulation of pathogenic bacteria in the small intestine; otherwise known as small intestinal bacterial overgrowth (which can also occur due to insufficient gastric acid); and intestinal viruses or parasites will also cause inflammation, as can hormone imbalances. Auto-immune diseases such as Crohn's disease, celiac disease, diverticulitis, and uncontrolled diabetes can also damage the microvilli and allow leakages to develop.

Leaky gut can vary in severity from displaying very few symptoms when there is only minor inflammation to being very severe when leaky gut is combined with an overgrowth of pathogens. This can lead to a potentially serious condition called endotoxemia, which causes systemic inflammation, increased inflammatory cytokines, and activation of inflammatory immune cells throughout the whole body. For this reason, anyone suffering from multiple chronic inflammatory symptoms should first consult a functional or integrative medical professional to be assessed for leaky gut and possible endotoxemia rather than accept prescriptions of potentially toxic medications.

Pathogenic bacteria in the small intestine produce excess methane and hydrogen gases, which can be detected easily through a simple breath test. Leaky gut and small intestinal bacterial overgrowth are extraordinarily complex conditions; if you suspect you may have either condition, I strongly encourage you to seek advice from a qualified professional experienced in treating these conditions.

As we reach the final stage of digestion, we encounter the area with the most significant colony of microbes, the large intestine, which houses the 'rainforest within' discussed earlier. The diversity of microbes in your large intestine directly reflects the diversity of plant food in your diet. Those of an allergic nature who are forced to eat restricted diets due to necessary allergen avoidance can inadvertently reduce their microbial diversity, which results in increased food intolerances. This is due to a reduction in the bacterial pathways these microbes make available to digest various foods and is another reason why the Allergic March occurs. Patients develop increasing numbers of food sensitivities due to their inability to digest them properly.

If you suffer from persistent and repeated gut distress, such as diarrhoea, constipation, bloating, gas, or heartburn, these will increase the stress levels in your body and consequently impact the severity of eczema, whether from the stress cycles covered in the next chapter or malabsorption of nutrients. Due to the complexity of the gut system and the number of organs involved in the digestion, absorption, and elimination processes, if it is apparent that something is amiss here, I highly recommend working with a functional medical practitioner to correct your gut function.

Our eczema spider now shows how gut function, including our microbiome, influences and ties to all the other legs of the eczema spider. You have learnt how having an impaired gut function increases nutritional deficiencies, which can lead to having a dry, dysfunctional skin barrier, a decreased ability to detoxify, increased stress, negative impacts on the immune and allergic states, suppression of your ability to carry out DNA instructions, and consequently, a detrimental effect on the health of your skin.

In the next chapter, I will explain one of the most common eczema complaints, "Why do I get Eczema flares when I am stressed?" This is a very interesting and revealing part of the spider web, with even more cycles to expose.

Your action points for this chapter are on the following page.

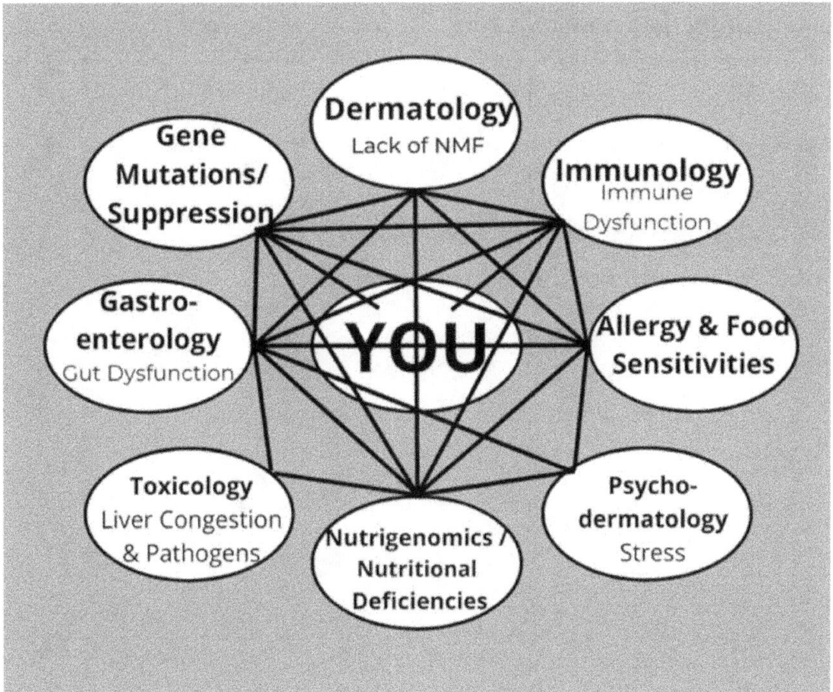

Action points

1. Avoid unnecessary antibiotic exposure, including food preservatives, meat from antibiotic-fed animals, drinking chlorinated water, and eating foods contaminated with pesticides. Research and seek advice regarding natural antibiotics to use for infections.

2. Avoid non-steroidal anti-inflammatory painkiller medications and instead transition to natural forms of pain relief while seeking to resolve the issues causing pain.

3. In pregnancy and childbirth, aim for a natural vaginal birth and breastfeed for at least six months. If a C-section is necessary, request the baby is swabbed with vaginal fluid (so long as there are no known infections present that could put your baby at risk). In case of C-section, inability to breastfeed, or if the mother received intravenous antibiotics during labour, the baby should be given infant probiotics mixed into a little sterilised water to manipulate the microbiome towards better health.

4. Eat food as close to nature as possible, preferably fresh, organic, unprocessed, and home-prepared. Avoid artificial additives, including colours and flavour enhancers.

5. Add anaerobically fermented foods to your diet.

6. Reduce stress.

7. Exercise regularly.

8. Take premium broad-spectrum probiotics.

11

The Stress Connection

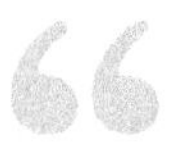 *Run! There are terrorists with knives!"*

Before we moved overseas as missionaries, I took one of my daughters out to the Boxing Day sales at our local shopping mall in the United Kingdom. While walking through the centre of the mall, we suddenly heard a male voice shouting in an urgent guttural roar. Although we could not understand what he was shouting, he sounded highly fearful. As we turned to look behind in the direction of the voice, people began to run towards us, their faces in a perfect expression of terror. I froze, clutching my young daughter's hand, trying to ascertain what was happening. Then a man ran past, his face etched with panic, and he yelled at me in a primal scream, "Run! There are terrorists with knives!"

I did not need a second instruction. I suddenly experienced a burst of energy, and my mental alertness rose to new heights. At superfast speed, I assessed my options for either hiding or escaping, made my decision, and told my daughter we had to run. We turned and fled towards the main doors at the entrance to the mall. I had read stories of terrorist ambushes where shooters were waiting to mow down those running from the building. I did not know if that would be the case. There were many people ahead of us. I figured we could head to the nearest door and listen for any gunfire or screaming. I could not hear either. Thus, I considered the doors still our safest option. As we ran past the escalator, crowds were piling onto it from the upper floors, with everyone attempting to vacate as quickly as possible. One man decided on a faster option and leapt over the side rail, landing heavily on the floor below before scrambling to his feet and dashing for the door. We ran past abandoned empty buggies and shopping bags that had been thrown into shop doorways, the just-purchased merchandise no longer considered valuable compared to saving your life. It was every man for himself, and everyone was trying to escape.

When we reached the automatic double doors, to my dismay, they were broken and had been sealed shut. Only one single glass exit door remained available, which was crammed full of panicking people desperately trying to push and squeeze their way through to safety. I yelled at my daughter to slip through their legs and told her to run down the street to a particular store, informing her I would meet her there. At that point, I wanted to get her out of there, and her holding my hand while I was stuck behind the adult traffic jam was keeping her inside in the panic. Finally, I burst through the door and ran faster than I had run in years, down the street to the muster point I had told her about. We were safe. We both started to shake. We had used all our energy supplies to flee, and both felt physically exhausted. As much as we wanted to go home, I did not want my daughter to grow up with a phobia of malls, so we stayed in the area until the police returned order, and everything looked normal again. Then I took her back to the mall, where we sat down to drink hot chocolate and eat a treat. I wanted to help alleviate the bad memory with a more pleasant one. It was not terrorists after all, but two rival gangs who had decided to fight in the mall with swords, causing total pandemonium.

I share this story because it illustrates the 'fight or flight' response in the body very well. When you read this, it is easy to relate; you know how you would feel if you were in that situation with your young child, especially as we live in a time where terrorist assaults, mass shootings, and violent attacks are seen in the news all too often. Subconsciously, we are on higher alert for these things because this threat has become a sad part of life.

One of the most common questions clients ask me is: "Why does stress aggravate eczema?" I will answer this in this chapter as we examine how stress impacts eczema.

People who suffer from eczema typically display higher stress levels than those with healthy skin, and periods of heightened stress commonly cause eczema to flare up more. Studies conducted on children with eczema show a direct correlation between the severity of their symptoms and their stress levels. Investigations also found that children who suffer from eczema display different emotional responses than children without eczema. For example, they typically display increased fear responses and anxiety (most likely, adults with eczema do as well, but the study did not include them). As a result, scientists and medics have often questioned, like another chicken and egg scenario, which came first? Did eczema cause elevated stress, or does high stress cause eczema?

The scientists conducting the study stated they were unsure what the answer to that question was. (16) Personally, now that I have developed the Eczemology™ map, I believe it can be both a cause of flares and a consequence, depending on where a person is entangled in the eczema spider web. However, it is highly unlikely that eczema would develop solely from stress alone, without other cofactors being involved, such as microbiome dysbiosis.

Anyone with eczema knows that emotionally stressful events trigger flare-ups and the deterioration of eczema symptoms in their skin. However, chronic stress has also been shown to affect the eczema risk in the next generation. For example, when examining stress associations with eczema, it was found that the children of parents who were engaged in relational conflicts were found to have a markedly higher risk of developing eczema. (16) This is likely to be the result of the impact of the mother's stress response on her gut microbiome, which results in the baby being born with gut dysbiosis and then predisposed to eczema development. The effects on the gut are just one of the ways that stress impacts eczema.

Stress is a necessary part of life. Not all stress is detrimental, just as not all inflammation is detrimental. There is such a thing as good stress. When striving to achieve something, the boost of stress hormones enables us to get things done more efficiently. When the project is completed, we are rewarded with endorphins and dopamine as we celebrate our success. However, there is another form of stress response that occurs due to perceived threats, which is designed to help facil-itate our survival. This switches on what is called our 'fight or flight' response.

During that Boxing Day event, we experienced a perceived threat to our survival. This resulted in the release of cortisol and adrenaline, the stress hormones. They cause numerous reactions in the body. First-ly, they cause the liver to release the glucose stores that have been reserved for times when emergency energy is needed. This gives us a sudden rush of energy and enables us to fight with extra strength or run faster than normal to facilitate escape. It can also enable us to think more clearly to assess the situation before us. However, some people have a fear response that shuts down the prefrontal cortex of their brain (responsible for learning and memory), which causes that mind-gone-blank scenario where they cannot reason effectively to determine what to do.

Simultaneous to this energy dump is the shutting down of any process-es that are not immediately necessary for survival. Things like healing and digestion are not essential at that moment and are temporarily postponed, diverting more energy to the muscles and cardiovascular system, where it is needed more urgently. Cortisol and adrenaline also suppress the innate immune system and the production of stomach acid and enzymes. Let's face it, regardless of how tasty they smell, I really was not likely to stop and buy a pretzel while trying to flee from a perceived terrorist attack. When these processes occur in response to a short-term threat, they are helpful. They help us resolve the issue, and then we can return to normal afterwards and recover our equilibrium. However, problems start to occur when we do not return to normal, and our stress levels remain elevated for long periods.

In the case of eczema, suppression of innate immunity caused by high levels of stress allows the pathogenic bacteria to flourish on the skin, which in turn causes increased inflammation. We covered this in Chapter 7. As the pathogens increase, they start to invade below the skin barrier. The disturbed keratinocyte skin cells release thymic stro-mal lymphopoietin and trigger the cascade of immune responses, the waking up of naïve dendritic cells, the resulting Th2 dominance, and the class switching of B cells to IgE antibody production leading to an increased allergic response.

This reduction in the innate immune response explains why the skin of eczema patients is frequently colonised with *Staphylococcus aureus*. Eczema patients live with abnormal levels of stress due to the nature of their illness as they try to live, sleep, and function in constant discomfort; therefore, the levels of innate protection in their skin are consistently suppressed. Consequently, they have higher levels of pathogens residing on their skin. Studies have shown a direct correlation between the number of resident *Staphylococci* bacteria on a person's skin and the severity of their eczema. In addition, other organisms such as yeast *Malassezia furfur* or *molluscum contagiosum virus* are seen more regularly in the skin of eczema patients than in the skin of healthy people. Studies have also shown a link to attention deficiency hyperactive disorder in children with eczema, although this inability to focus may well be due to their constant itching and sleep deprivation. (16)

As we saw in Chapter 7, in addition to stress reducing the immunity of the skin, the resulting Th2 dominance leads to the release of cytokines that inhibit the expression of genes on the epidermal differentiation complex portion of chromosome 1, which are necessary to produce S100 skin proteins (e.g., filaggrin). This leads to the inability to produce new healthy skin and creates a cycle of eczema causing stress, and stress causing eczema.

The other major system that is suppressed in times of stress is the digestive system, especially the production of stomach acid and digestive enzymes. This is supposed to be temporary to redirect the energy for digestion to immediate survival, after which we should recover our equilibrium as things reset back to normal. We humans have never been able to carry stress for long periods. It burdens the body in many ways and is one of the reasons why Jesus likened us to sheep in the Bible. If you load a sheep with burdens, it will just lay down under the weight. They are not beasts of burden, and neither are we. When stress becomes chronic, and the digestive system is suppressed for extended periods, gut dysbiosis can occur. Suppression of stomach acid means we will be unable to dissolve the food we ingest properly. In addition, the acidity levels will not be high enough to sterilise the food by killing harmful bacteria. These bacteria will then pass into the small intestine, which is the perfect temperature for them to flourish and proliferate, creating gut dysbiosis (an imbalance of good and bad microbes). This will contribute to nutritional deficiencies as the gut will lack the necessary pathways from the commensurate or friendly microbes to break down and synthesise all the nutrients in the diet. As we saw in the previous chapter, these deficiencies further impact the ability to produce the skin proteins and enzymes necessary for a healthy epidermal barrier. Therefore, the skin continues to form in a manner predisposed to eczema along with the resulting immune and allergy cycles. (Nutritional deficiencies also cause a host of other health issues outside the scope of this book).

In addition to the nutritional side, gut dysbiosis also leads to an inability to produce the compounds needed to manufacture neurotransmitters such as serotonin and gamma-aminobutyric acid; the gut microbes are the primary producers of these neurotransmitters. A deficiency in these short-chain fatty acids will detrimentally impact our feelings of peace, leading to increased anxiety and depression, which further heightens stress levels and sets yet another cycle in motion.

The chart on the following page is a visual representation of the impact of stress on eczema.

Now that you can see how stress impacts eczema, the question you will no doubt want to ask is: "What can you do about it?" There are seven main areas of stress that we need to address. You may not suffer from them all, but as you read through them, you should be able to identify the ones that do impact you. You can then work on those areas to reduce your stress impact.

HOW STRESS AFFECTS ECZEMA

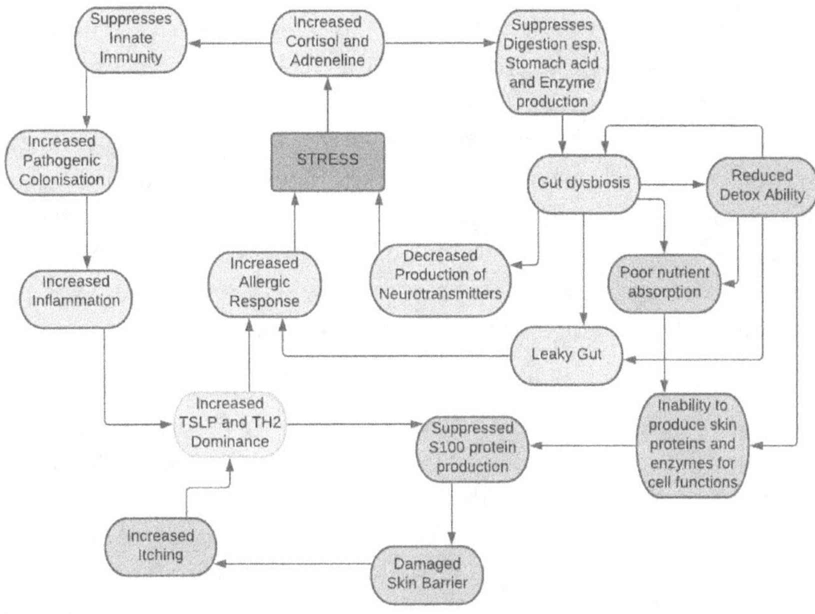

1. Inflammatory Stress

2. Sleep Stress

3. Emotional Stress

4. Nutritional Stress

5. Gastrointestinal Stress

6. Cellular Stress

7. Spiritual Stress

1. Inflammatory Stress

Inflammation, as we have already discussed, occurs during times of injury and illness to bring more cells to the area to resolve an issue. It also happens in response to strenuous exercise. (23) The whole point of inflammation is to repair damage. Therefore, sustaining any injury will cause the body to release inflammatory cytokines, which recruit immune cells to help clear the damage and repair the tissue.

The purpose of exercise is to build health and fitness; however, particularly in the case of strength or endurance training, this is achieved by putting muscles under duress. When we subject our muscles to microscopic tears by exercising intensely, the body responds with inflammation to repair the damage and reinforce the muscle. The repeated tearing and repairing build up the muscles and causes them to increase in size and strength. As part of this rebuilding cycle, the cells produce inflammatory cytokines to recruit cells for muscle repair. As the inflammatory process gets underway, it is common to experience delayed onset muscle soreness, otherwise known as DOMS, the next day, often peaking around 48 hours after exercise.

Regardless of whether inflammation is caused by injury, exercise, chronic illness, or otherwise, as we saw in Chapter 7, the area floods with immune cells and inflammatory cytokines. The unfortunate downside of this for eczema patients is that the influx will also bring areas of skin damage to the attention of those cells, causing increased inflammation in areas affected by eczema. This also happens when blood vessels dilate to allow the body to cool down during exercise. As a result, the immune cells are bought closer to the skin's surface, allowing them to identify pathogens on and in the skin. This partially answers another question I am frequently asked about eczema: "Why does eczema flare up during or after exercise?"

Further to this question, Salty sweat can also irritate eczema when exercising, so exercise with a fan or other cooling system to limit sweating if this affects you, and shower immediately afterwards to minimise the irritation. In addition, chemical or petroleum-based emollients block the pores and cause the sweat to build up under the skin instead of being released through the pores. This causes the sweat to leech into the surrounding tissues, disturbing the keratinocyte cells and triggering an immune response to the sweat itself. Studies have shown that many eczema patients have developed an allergy to their own sweat as a result.

We have already covered how to reduce inflammation in Chapter 7, and the same tactics will work for inflammatory stress. Ginger, curcumin from turmeric, frankincense, omega-3 oils, and probiotics have all been shown to be effective at reducing the levels of inflammation in the body by various mechanisms and, in some cases, increasing the cytokines that reduce inflammation. (12, 13, 23, 24, 77, 78, 82)

2. Sleep Stress

Insufficient, interrupted, and poor-quality sleep have been shown to increase inflammation in the body, with different forms of sleep deprivation causing different reactions. (79, 80, 81)

Our bodies function best when we operate within our circadian rhythm. This is the natural waking cycle triggered by ultraviolet light from the sun and the natural progression towards sleep triggered by the sunlight reducing from dusk to evening. With the invention of electric lighting, we have lost the natural lighting cycle we would have previously responded to and now subject ourselves to constant blue light sources that mimic the sun's rays and throw our circadian rhythm off balance. We often spend our evenings watching things online, working on our laptops, reading e-books, and catching up on social media. We also light our houses with bright lighting far into the night; even when we do finally retire, our bedrooms are invaded by light from outside sources such as traffic or street lighting. All this exposure interrupts the circadian rhythm and affects our ability to produce the melatonin needed to induce feelings of tiredness and to sleep well enough to harness the healing effects of our rest. Interruption of the circadian rhythm has been shown to increase TNF-α and C-reactive protein levels, both of which are indicative of increased inflammation. (81)

Sleep deprivation, whether from consistent late nights and early mornings or from having your sleep disrupted either by your own or your child's itching eczema, is another cause of sleep stress. Studies have shown that being deprived of sleep or having your sleep constantly disrupted increase cortisol levels in the blood and lead to impaired stress responses. (79, 80) We have already established that high levels of cortisol and stress hormones impact both the inflammatory response and digestive capability, so we must be careful to protect our sleep quality as much as feasibly possible. We can support our circadian rhythm with some simple but effective measures.

Straightforward steps such as activating the blue light filters on phones and electronic devices and turning down light sources by using dimmed lamps instead of full ceiling lights in the evening will help to restore the natural brain rhythms for sleep and wakefulness cycles. We can also use blackout curtains or eye masks to provide much greater darkness during our sleeping hours. Children, in particular, benefit from using blue light filters and restricting using electronic devices at least 2 hours before bedtime.

A brisk walk in the early morning sunshine will help to improve our wakefulness, helping to restore the 'wake' part of the cycle. Weather permitting, I take a 1-mile walk every morning. If for some reason, it is not possible, I will stand outside on the porch and take some deep breaths of air while stretching instead. It is still natural light and intentional movement.

Toward the evening, as well as dimming the lighting and limiting the use of electronic devices (or using blue light filters), another evening walk in the dusk or later light will help to trigger the 'sleep' side of the circadian rhythm. In addition, consider checking your vitamin B6 status, as it is necessary to produce melatonin. Tryptophan, an amino acid, also helps to produce better quality sleep. (Have you noticed how you feel sleepy after eating the roast turkey dinner at Thanksgiving or Christmas? You can thank the tryptophan in the turkey and the vitamin B6 in the potatoes for that.) Personally, I find I experience much better sleep when I drink a protein shake containing tryptophan around an hour before I retire. I also keep my room very dark, and my phone has the blue light filter permanently switched on, even throughout the day.

Sleep can also be disrupted by nasal swellings such as polyps or sleep apnea. Being unable to breathe properly through the nose will necessitate mouth breathing, which has been shown to decrease sleep quality. Sleep apnea also disrupts sleep and can be potentially dangerous as breathing repeatedly stops and starts throughout the night. Constantly waking up feeling exhausted or snoring loudly could be symptoms of sleep apnea. Seek advice regarding this if it applies to you.

Many other health conditions can affect sleep quality. For example, uncontrolled or undiagnosed diabetes can cause excessive thirst and urination, leading to frequent waking for water and consequent bathroom trips. Mineral deficiencies can cause painful leg cramps at night, jarring sleepers awake in sudden agony as they fly out of bed trying to loosen the tight ball in their calf muscle. (Yes, I have been there too, but I resolved this with magnesium supplementation.) If you constantly wake feeling tired or struggle to maintain quality sleep throughout the night, I recommend you examine why and consider seeking advice and perhaps tests to rule out or uncover any undiagnosed medical conditions.

3. Emotional Stress

Another issue affecting our emotions is the constant availability of never-ending, stress-inducing news stories. Before the advent of online activities, we only really knew about the events in our local vicinity. Our local bank may have been robbed, a car accident may have happened on the main road, or some other newsworthy event may have occurred to trigger an emotional response. However, this would have been the odd occasion, not the norm. Fast forward to today, and we hear a constant stream of stress-inducing news from every part of the globe: tsunamis, volcanic eruptions, earthquakes, terrorist attacks, kidnaps, rapes, murders, child abuse, and corruption scandals. The list is never-ending. Sitting down and watching the news during downtime may be relaxing, but this is not helping our stress response. We struggle to reclaim equilibrium when constantly exposing our brains and emotions to stress-inducing news stories.

Our brains are extraordinarily complex; however, despite this, studies have shown that our brains are easily fooled by our emotions. They cannot tell the difference between what is real and what is not. Hence why you can experience real fear responses when watching a scary movie or why it is so effective to visualise yourself in great scenarios, such as confidently speaking on stage or imagining celebrating the achievement of a goal before you have even accomplished it. For the same reason, constantly subjecting ourselves to violence and threat from news stories, computer games, or even cyberbullying on social media can cause our brains to feel we are at risk, to trigger our 'fight or flight' response, and to release unnecessary cortisol and adrenaline. A healthy individual without chronic inflammatory disease may not notice any issues with these, but those who are trying to establish a healthier stress response and reduce their inflammation should consider what they expose themselves to. You do not need to be unnecessarily elevating your stress hormones and inflammatory cytokines when trying to heal eczema.

Unresolved trauma also affects our stress response. We may feel that we have moved on when we bury emotionally painful experiences and refuse to think about them, but they are still working their insidious effects within our subconscious mind. Past traumas can lead to higher stress levels due to increased fear responses. On an extreme level, people who have been victims of some form of violent attack or traumatic event may find themselves consciously avoiding similar situations; for example, no longer wanting to frequent shopping malls after a perceived terrorist incident, avoiding lifts after being stuck in one, avoiding particular forms of transport after being involved in an accident, or even avoiding eating out after bad experiences from allergic cross-contamination. These types of decisions may seem like we are just exercising wisdom or our personal preference, but on many occasions, the avoidance is due to a subconscious survival mechanism operating from unresolved emotional stress linked to the incident.

Similarly, experiences such as past rejection, bullying, shaming, and abuse can leave emotional scars that need to be resolved. These types of emotional stress can work silently in the background, sabotaging what we are trying to achieve in life because, subconsciously, we still believe we are somehow of lower worth than others. For example, if you have been bullied or constantly experienced rejection, you could easily develop a perfectionist mentality because you were never accepted for being yourself. Therefore, you may now feel that you must produce results far superior to everyone else to be accepted as equal. Or perhaps your dreams and aspirations constantly elude you regardless of how hard you work because your subconscious psyche still remembers how no one wanted to pick you for any team activities, leaving you the last one on the sidelines feeling rejected year in, year out; you may still believe that no-one will pick you for that contract, sale, presentation, etc. As silent and unnoticed as they are, these unresolved emotional conflicts cause additional stress in our lives, whether pushing us towards perfectionism just to feel remotely good enough or destroying our self-confidence whenever we want to step out and do something. The frustration of not being able to achieve can be real and noticeable. However, the stress that results from the unresolved wrong beliefs about ourselves and our abilities can be working away in the dark without us knowing. All this elevated stress can then impact our digestion and immune function too.

The blue zones we spoke of earlier thrive partly due to their close-knit families and communities. They tend to have strong social bonds and supportive networks. Community is essential for well-being, which is why solitary confinement was developed as a form of torture by oppressive regimes. Humans thrive in encouraging fellowship and interaction with many documented benefits, such as an improved sense of well-being, reduced depression, and immune function. Conversely, living with abuse or relationship conflict will also affect your health but in a detrimental manner. If you are living in a situation that is physically or emotionally harmful to your health, you need to give yourself permission to leave and move to a safe place where you can give yourself space to heal. There are emotional and physical support organisations in your local area that can assist if this is the case. You must remove yourself from danger and get the appropriate help. Sometimes the situation has already ended, but the anger at the offence is still very raw, and the resentment continues to eat away inside.

Lewes B. Smedes wonderfully stated: "To forgive is to set a prisoner free and discover that the prisoner was you." Forgiveness does not excuse the wrong that was committed against you. It just sets you free from living in the past, constantly hoping they will get their just recompense. We cannot travel forward if we are constantly looking in the rearview mirror. If you think about those who have perpetrated evil against you, they have most likely moved on with their lives and never even consider what their actions cost you. It is you, not them, who is held bound by the emotional conflict inside. Forgiveness releases you from being tied to the event. Consider the following quote from Jesus in the Bible; when He had been crucified and was hanging in immense pain on the cross, He prayed: "Father, forgive them for they know not what they do." I have found it easier to forgive people when I remember that I have not lived in their shoes. I have not walked their life or experienced the struggles and abuse that they may have experienced. One thing I tell my children when they are hurt by someone else's actions is that: "Hatred is not something we are born with. It is something we are taught." An old friend once told me, "Hurt people, hurt people." It is a succinct way to say that those who have hidden unresolved hurts inadvertently end up hurting others. It is so true. Forgive and pray that the offender will find healing from whatever trauma caused them to become that way, then put them in the hands of God and remove yourself from the equation for the sake of your health.

Although there is so much more I can say about emotional stress, including the stress that comes from grief, financial failures, divorce, job losses, sickness, and many more, this book is about eczema, not psychology or counselling. So I will leave it at this point here. However, as I have already pointed out, stress detrimentally impacts your immune response and healing ability. Thus, if something I have mentioned has exposed any hidden wounds, I strongly encourage you to seek appropriate counselling to find closure on unresolved emotional conflicts.

4. Nutritional Stress

We have already spoken about nutrition in Chapter 10. If the body does not have sufficient nutrients to facilitate its necessary functions, it will experience stress and disease as a result. Nutritional deficiencies also impact our emotional stress as a lack of fermentable fibres will equate to an insufficiency of short-chain fatty acids, which are required to produce neurotransmitters for brain and emotional health. This creates a cycle in which nutritional deficiencies create stress. Stress then reduces the digestive capability, which leads to nutritional deficiencies and an inability to detoxify properly, causing more stress. We can mitigate nutritional stress by loving and supporting ourselves with the right nutritionally dense foods and additional supplements, as necessary. As I said before, your life is precious. You are worth every penny.

5. Gastrointestinal Stress

I previously spoke about the microbiome and gut health in Chapter 10. Unresolved issues in any area of the gut and digestive tract can also cause gastrointestinal stress. Digestion starts in the brain, not the gut, and you really need to look from the top down to assess where any problems originate. In the previous chapter, I briefly explained the digestion process and the most common causes of gastrointestinal stress. It is important to review these and assess if your gut health is contributing to your stress load and, if so, to take corrective action to rectify it.

6. Cellular Stress

Oxidative stress is one of the major problems associated with atopic dermatitis. (76) We have already spoken of the problems created by unstable molecules; however, there is another aspect of losing electrons to oxidisation. Oxidation also affects our body's magnetic charge, or polarity, which increases oxidative stress.

Electrons are negatively charged, so when we lose them through oxidation, we become more positively charged. This also affects the communication channels of cells, as 'messages' are often passed along an electron chain from one electron to the next. If electrons are missing, it can lead to aborted or inefficient instructions in much the same way as loss of function mutations lead to an inability to produce proteins effectively.

I previously spoke of the importance of managing free radicals and oxidation. Your diet is one of the most effective ways for you to take control of this. However, there is another highly effective way to reduce oxidation, regain lost electrons, and restore the correct polarity of the body. This is called grounding.

Scientific studies have shown that being in contact with the surface of the Earth, for example, by walking barefoot on soil or sand, causes the body to receive additional free electrons from the ground. This restabilises our molecules and acts as another powerful form of antioxidant. Scientists observed remarkable improvements in immune function, healing of resistant sores, improved sleep, normalisation of the day and night cortisol rhythm, reduced pain, reduced stress, increased heart rate variability, improved blood flow, and the switching of the nervous system from the 'fight or flight' response (sympathetic) back to 'equilibrium and healing' (parasympathetic) activity. (86)

The benefits of grounding begin after only 15 minutes of walking barefoot on the beach or grass. I admit that not everyone wants to, or can, walk outside barefoot. Still, thankfully, there are now a variety of grounding systems available that allow prolonged or repeated contact with the Earth, even from inside your home. These mats and bedsheets have cords that connect with the Earth, either via a grounded wall outlet or being attached to a ground rod that touches the Earth outside a window, for example. They then provide simple conductive systems that allow a person to pick up the free electrons from the Earth without being outside barefoot. Indeed, they can be used whilst sleeping, working at a desk, or standing in the kitchen cooking. Grounding footwear is also available, which has conductive plugs in the soles of the shoes and allows constant grounding while worn.

Another source of cellular stress is mitochondrial dysfunction. Scientists used to teach that the mitochondria were like the batteries of our cells; however, they are much more than just batteries. Around 90% of our cellular energy is produced by the mitochondria in our cells, which convert the energy from our food into the ATP energy needed for our cellular functions. If mitochondria are functioning at sub-optimal levels, this will result in them having a reduced capacity for producing ATP. Consequently, our cells will lack the energy to carry out their functions efficiently, which can lead to intense fatigue. (65)

A growing number of studies have revealed that mitochondrial dysfunction can lead to various diseases, from diabetes to Parkinson's and rare genetic diseases.

The DNA of our mitochondria are bacterial in nature, which means they are harmed by antibiotic exposure, toxins, heavy metals, and herbicides and pesticides such as glyphosate. This is extremely important as it links back to our stress response involving the Vagus nerve.

Stress affects the Vagus nerve as it switches on what we know as the 'fight or flight' response. However, some scientists have now realised there is a third stress response that switches on if we can neither take fight nor flee. This is the play dead or freeze response. In the short term, this is like a deer that freezes in the headlights of an oncoming car. However, when this type of inescapable stress happens over the long term, it can cause our cells to go into a type of hibernation state.

The brain, Vagus nerve, and cells all communicate with each other. When the brain is stressed, the Vagus nerve can become subdued. Dr Stephen Porges, an eminent psychiatrist, developed the Porges theory that the Vagus nerve has two sides – the dorsal and ventral sides. When all is well, we operate on the ventral side, but when there has been trauma, crises, or long-term stress, the Vagus nerve can start operating on the dorsal side. This subdues the activity of the mitochondria in the cells, diverting energy from ATP production to cellular defence and survival. Essentially, it tells the cells that because you are under perceived threat and can neither fight nor flee, they need to go into a siege mentality, to conserve as much energy as possible, and instead divert what they do have to defence tactics like putting up thicker shields around your cell walls. Unfortunately, this means your energy production is severely depressed, as are all your cellular functions, such as producing enzymes and following DNA instructions, along with your ability to receive nutrients into your cells. Cellular processes can become so suppressed that people physically struggle to get out of bed or do anything because they are too exhausted. They can also display symptoms of nutritional deficiencies, even if they have been eating well, as their cells cannot take up and utilise the nutrients effectively. If we overdo activity and exert ourselves too much over a long period, we can trigger this same effect. If it lasts only for a short time, it is useful and our body's way of telling us to stop, rest and recuperate. But if we get stuck on dorsal Vagal function because the stressful events have either been too huge or too prolonged, this can lead to many illnesses such as chronic fatigue syndrome, myalgic encephalomyelitis (ME), and post-traumatic stress disorder, in addition to scenarios when you know you are whacked out and clearly unwell, but your doctors are telling you there is nothing wrong, and all your tests are normal.

This whole process also works vice versa. If the mitochondria become stressed, say from toxins, antibiotics, or nutritional deficiencies. They communicate to the Vagus nerve to depress function to lower activity to conserve fuel for danger mitigation. The connections and communication ability between our brain, Vagus nerve, and mitochondria explain why emotional and cellular stress are closely related. Unresolved emotional conflicts or long-term stressful situations put the body into the 'play dead' conservation state. This then suppresses digestion and immune function. It quickly becomes another whole cycle by itself.

Electrical Vagal nerve stimulation has been proven to heal chronic illnesses by reactivating the ventral side of the Vagus nerve. However, as most of us do not have expensive nerve-stimulating equipment lying around at home, you will be happy to know there are alternative, effective ways to stimulate the Vagus nerve ourselves. Actions that raise the heart rate promote peace and tranquillity. Laughter and joy, benevolence and kindness, all stimulate Vagal activity and send messages to the brain that all is well, we are no longer under threat, and we can focus on healing and energy production again. Hence, we can help turn off our inflammatory response by doing things that communicate wellness to our bodies. What kinds of things? Laughing out loud, singing at the top of your voice, meditating, getting sufficient high-quality sleep, spending time enjoying the company of loved ones, playing fun games with the kids or your pets, and getting involved in benevolence or charitable activities.

Regardless of the type of stress, in addition to finding ways to mitigate stress, there are some common all-round remedies that are beneficial. Firstly, taking magnesium is essential as we use magnesium for over 300 biochemical reactions in the body, including enzyme reactions involved in making S100 proteins. All types of stress, whether physical or emotional, have been proven to deplete magnesium from the body. Magnesium deficiency then decreases the ability to overcome the stress from these situations, which compounds the problem. (87) Therefore, taking a high-quality magnesium supplement is essential for eczema sufferers to mitigate the depletion caused by the chronic stress of their skin discomfort. Otherwise, the resulting deficiency leaves eczema suffers with a reduced ability to cope with the other stressors that occur in life. Here are some additional supplements that have been shown to be helpful in reducing the impact of stress:

- **Alpha-linolenic acid** from flax and chia seeds (2 tbsp of each) can help support mitochondrial function, relieve oxidative stress, and assist in removing excess heavy metals from the body.

- **L-carnitine** supplements have been shown to reverse age-related mitochondrial decline and many disease symptoms when taken at doses of up to 2 g daily. L-carnitine naturally occurs in red meat but also in other meats, albeit at lower levels.

- **Co-enzyme Q10** is a potent antioxidant that affects gene expression and cell signalling. It is found in the highest concentrations in organ meats, but for those who would rather not eat organs, it can also be safely supplemented up to 600 mg/day in divided doses. (66) (Co-enzyme Q10 does interact with Warfarin medication, so if you are taking any blood thinners or have any other medical conditions, you should seek professional advice from a qualified functional nutritionist.)

- **Nicotinamide adenine dinucleotide** is involved in over 200 cellular redox reactions and over 4000 enzyme reactions. We can make it from Niacin (vitamin B3), but it is also present in meat, the highest quantity being in liver. We can also make it from the amino acid tryptophan, which is found in meat, especially turkey. We can also obtain it by supplementing with Niacin or niacinamide (the no-flush version). (67)

- **Membrane phospholipids.** Taking supplements of 200–500 mg daily of essential fatty acids has been shown to result in the replacement of damaged membrane phospholipids with undamaged and unoxidised lipids, restoring mitochondrial function. Membrane phospholipids are found naturally in eicosapentaenoic acid and docosahexaenoic acid (EPA and DHA) from oily fish, krill oil, and alpha-linolenic acid from plants, e.g., flax and chia seeds. (68)

- **L-threonine** is a natural phytochemical found in green leaves that has been shown to reduce physiological and phycological stress responses. Dramatically increasing your dietary intake of green leafy vegetables would also likely reap the same benefits. (114)

Essential oils can also be used to reduce stress and induce feelings of calm. My go-to resource for essential oil preparations and recipe blends is '**The Complete Book of Essential Oils and Aromatherapy**' by Valerie Ann Wormwood. She advises oils such as lavender, geranium, rosemary, and many others to help calm the emotions and the stress response. They can be added to diffusers or diluted in carrier oils and used as body moisturisers. Lavender is particularly effective; I have even used it to calm my dog when he was terrified by the terrifically loud thunderclaps in Trinidad.

Adaptogenic herbs are also an extremely useful addition to our arsenal. Rhodiola, ashwagandha, ginseng, schisandra, dong kwai, and astragalus are all commonly used to provide stress support. If you would like to add these medicinal herbs to your healthcare routine, I recommend you find a qualified herbalist who can advise you and provide clean sources of these herbs.

Meditation is another time-proven method to reduce stress. Articles have been published showing many beneficial alterations in immune function, gene expression, inflammation, and sense of well-being. (89) Although prayer and meditation are often spoken of together as if they are one and the same thing, they are markedly different. Prayer, particularly for the evangelical Christian, can often be waging spiritual warfare and is definitely not a form of relaxation. Meditation, however, is more of a mindfulness practice of sitting quietly and concentrating on breathing, becoming aware of our feelings and where our thoughts wander. Meditating can also be conducted using spiritual texts such as Bible verses, quietly and mindfully mulling over their meaning and how they apply to us personally. We can use our meditation time to visualise the results that we desire, such as clear and healed skin. With the benefits of meditating and mindfulness being shown to reduce inflammation, it is a tool that eczema patients should utilise to help reduce stress levels.

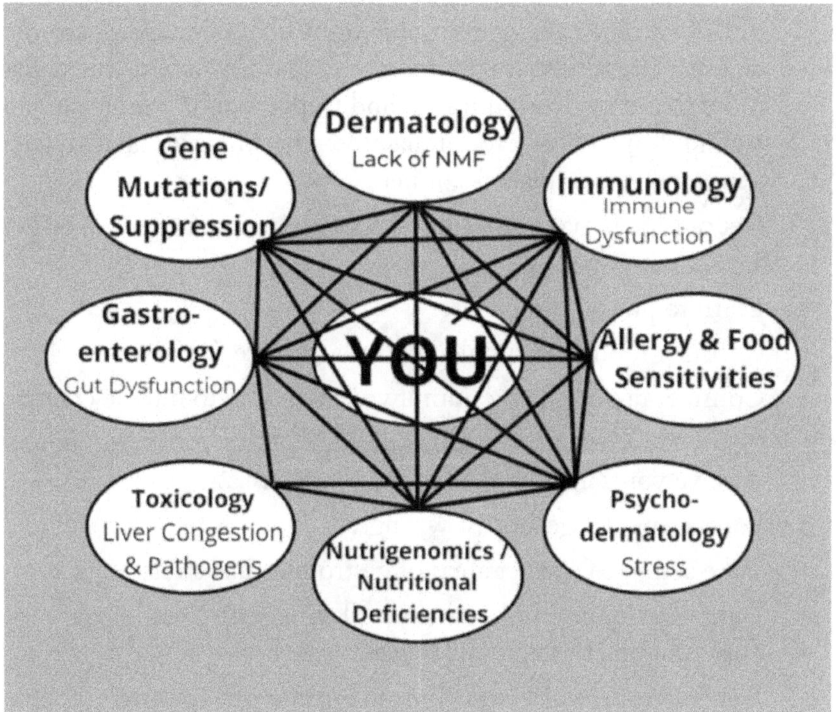

Our Eczema spider web is almost complete and now shows how stress not only affects the integrity of the skin but also lowers digestive capability, leading to or compounding nutritional deficiencies, which in turn increases cellular stress and toxicity due to reduced detoxifying ability. Elevated stress levels also suppress gene function, hindering your ability to produce S100 skin proteins effectively. Finally, if that is not bad enough, stress also suppresses immune function and increases susceptibility to infections and allergic responses.

The final spider leg in our eczema map is toxicity, where we will examine which toxins are proven to increase eczema development and severity, where your exposure comes from, and how you can protect yourself.

Action points

- Establish a correct circadian rhythm. Spend time outside in natural sunlight every morning and ensure you use dimmed lighting in the evening, along with blue light filters on any electronic devices. Use blackout curtains or eye masks when sleeping. Eat foods that contain vitamin B6 and tryptophan if you need help feeling sleepy. Check for undiagnosed health issues such as sleep apnea, polyps, or diabetes, if necessary.
- Get outside in nature, walk barefoot on the grass or sand, or get a grounding mat.
- Learn to pray and meditate.
- Consider foods and supplements that reduce stress.
- Consider taking magnesium if you are prone to muscle cramps.
- Work to reduce your stress exposure, resolve past traumas, and remove yourself from dangerous situations.
- Forgive and let go of past wrongs.
- Take action to correct areas of gastrointestinal stress.
- Laugh out loud, sing, spend time playing with friends and loved ones, and practice acts of benevolence.
- Build a community and find your tribe of supportive people (consider joining our community, find out more on our website EczemaAcademy.com).

12

Toxic Soup

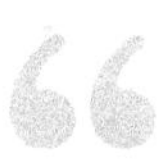

Embarking on a detox regime without first ensuring your detox pathways are working efficiently is, at best, a total waste of energy but, at worst, could be extremely harmful."

On a bright sunny afternoon in the United Kingdom many years ago, I looked out of the back patio doors to check on my friend's son playing in my backyard. He was certainly having fun, amusing himself by jumping on and off the manhole cover that sat squarely on our patio. Every time he landed heavily on the cover, a stream of brown liquid would shoot out high on each side, like a dirty fountain. At first, I was confused, wondering what was happening. Then it suddenly dawned on me. Under the manhole cover was the drainage system that led away the sewage from our property into the road to join the main sewage system. To my horror, I realised our drainage pipes must have become blocked, and he was innocently having a great time creating fountains of sewage every time he jumped onto the manhole cover. Needless to say, I quickly ended that game and found something else to occupy his time while my husband sought an emergency plumber to fix the drainage.

Some people ask why I leave toxins till last when other natural health medics look for toxicity first. To answer this, consider what happened with the sewage system at my house. Waste can only be removed if the drainage pipes are open. If the pipes are clogged, the waste will start to build up in the system and eventually either back up into your toilet again or leak out into some other place where it really does not belong, like it did in my backyard. Similarly, you must have open waste or detox pathways to detox the body safely. If your liver, kidneys, gallbladder, sweat mechanisms, and microbiome are not working optimally, when you embark on a detox, you will not be able to break down and eliminate the toxins released from your body. Consequently, they will back up into your bloodstream again, make you feel terrible, and then be reabsorbed into the fat and organs while your body attempts to detoxify by releasing these poisons through the skin, causing eczema to flare. Can you see that embarking on a detox regime without first ensuring your detox pathways are working efficiently is, at best, a total waste of energy but, at worst, could be extremely harmful?

Incorrect detoxing will affect the health of your skin and your gut, as many heavy metals interfere with skin processing, negatively impacting both the epidermis and the endothelial lining of the gut. The new toxin exposure will also increase systemic inflammation and allergic tendency. (59) In addition, if your diet and environment are not corrected, and you continue to fill your body with polluted foods and environmental toxins, you will add more toxicity and counteract any detox protocol. Nutritional deficiencies also increase toxicity as minerals are the primary agents to chelate or bind to the toxic metals, allowing them to be carried out of the body. Without them, we lack efficient chelation detox pathways. (60) Furthermore, if we are experiencing mitochondrial dysfunction or metabolic issues, for example, an underactive thyroid, these equate to our cells having less energy, which in turn means our detox organs are sluggish as they are made from those same cells. This also disrupts our ability to detox efficiently.

We must do things in the proper order. When the diet and the microbiome are improved, the primary environmental toxin exposures are minimised, and the liver, kidneys, and sweating detox pathways are opened and functioning correctly, ONLY THEN should we be looking to deal with the stored toxic overloads safely.

Before we look at ways to detox, I want to explain where the majority of our toxin exposures come from.

According to the Centers for Disease Control and Prevention, in 2019 alone, there were over 2.1 million cases of poison exposure in humans. Most of these were accidental poisonings, with surprisingly frequent occurrences resulting from people eating or drinking something they thought would benefit them. For example, people foraging for wild mushrooms or eating old potatoes with elevated levels of solanine. Poison control centres frequently publish warnings about the danger of repackaging chemicals into regular household containers, particularly recycled drink bottles. Unfortunately, many people, including children, have been killed or seriously injured from drinking chemicals that looked like apple juice or coloured soda drinks after they had been transferred into old soda or drinking water bottles for storage. It somehow seems even more tragic to be poisoned by something that a person expected to be good for them. Yet, we are exposed to chemicals every day, and similarly, many of them come in guises that we expect to be good for us.

The food we eat is often contaminated with invisible pesticides and herbicides; our cosmetics and personal hygiene products are laced with hidden toxins; our indoor furniture, furnishings, and decorating elements release harmful chemical gasses; ingredients and adjuvants used in pharmaceutical products and medical aids can be toxic; and the vehicles we use to drive around town pollute the air with exhaust fumes. Other chemicals leech into our environment and bodies from industrial pollutants, chemical cleaning agents, cigarette smoke from tobacco, processed foods full of preservatives, artificial colours and flavours, and chemical flavour enhancers. We can also be exposed to toxic heavy metal contamination from amalgam fillings, dental implants, prosthetic devices, and jewellery. Every day we can be exposed to thousands of chemical compounds before we have even finished breakfast.

There are already around 100,000 chemicals approved for use in the United States, and many of these are either known to be toxic, suspected of being toxic, or just have not been tested in any meaningful way to know if they are or not. Of those that are tested, most are examined only for whether they cause cancer when used in isolation; they are not tested for any other detrimental effects on the body, nor how their use may interact with other chemicals to increase their toxicity, either in the finished product or with other pollutants already stored in our bodies. Glyphosate is an excellent example of this. When combined with the other chemicals in Roundup™, researchers found that glyphosate was over 100 times **more** toxic than when tested in isolation.

Most people realise that overloading our bodies with toxins is not good for us. Still, eczema sufferers are also left wondering which or whether these toxins directly impact eczema development and severity. Much research has been conducted on this in recent years, especially since epidemiologists have noticed that the rate of eczema development has markedly increased over the last few decades. It correlates with increasing pollutant exposure, especially in urban areas. In addition, research has revealed that exposure to many individual toxins could influence the immune system during its development, specifically affecting the balance between Th1 and Th2 immune cell responses. This effect can be even more pronounced when toxins are combined. Therefore, let us look at the most common culprits known to affect eczema.

Air Pollution

Air pollution has been proven to be implicated in both the risk of developing eczema and the severity of eczema. We tend to think of air pollution as traffic fumes and smog; however, there are many more sources that are not only outside. Air contaminants can come from burning fossil fuels, traffic pollution, paints and solvents, adhesive fumes, off-gassing from furniture and furnishings, fumes from industrial power plants, tobacco smoke, mould and toxins, etc., to name a few. The air inside some buildings can expose you to more pollution than what exists in the environment outside, especially with modern construction methods, which lead to effectively sealed buildings lacking adequate ventilation to allow the pollution from the building process itself to reduce. We will discuss outside air pollution first.

Traffic pollution is the first and most apparent outdoor air pollutant, with many studies confirming its relevance to eczema development and severity.

In one study, eczema symptoms in 9–11-year-old children were shown to be significantly associated with exposure to benzene, PM10, nitrogen oxide compounds, and carbon monoxide, all of which are present in traffic pollution from vehicle exhaust fumes. (64) Benzene is also used to make plastics, resins, synthetic fibres, detergents, and some drugs and pesticides.

Another study in Taiwan showed similar results. A nationwide survey involving over 30,000 children demonstrated that the type of eczema affecting the more common flexural regions inside the elbows and at the back of the knees was positively associated with exposure to traffic-related air pollutants, which would have included those listed above. (90)

In Germany, a birth cohort study in an urban area showed strong positive relationships between the distance to the nearest main road and eczema development, with the most significant risk being for those living less than 50 meters away from busy streets. In addition, the study found that nitrogen dioxide exposure was positively associated with eczema, with scientists stating that their study "showed strong evidence that children exposed to ambient particular matter from traffic pollution have increased risk of developing atopic diseases and allergic sensitisation." (92) Several more studies have shown that outdoor air pollution influences the prevalence of atopic dermatitis.

Prenatal exposure to environmental pollutants is also associated with new infants developing atopic dermatitis and Th2-dominant immune systems. A study of 7030 children aged 6-13 demonstrated a positive correlation between atopic dermatitis and maternal smoking during pregnancy, in the first year after birth, or both. Furthermore, another study found that prenatal exposure to PM2.5 in combination with postnatal exposure to tobacco smoke increased the risk of eczema in infants. (97, 99) PM is an abbreviation for particulate matter, which is the term used to describe microscopic droplets of solid and liquid that are suspended in the air. These droplets are so minuscule that they can be inhaled easily and cause profound health implications. The number (e.g.,2.5) denotes the size of the particle in micrometres (e.g., 1000th of a millimetre). Hence PM2.5 is particulate matter consisting of droplets measuring only 0.0025 of a millimetre. To clarify, the second study assessed not only the infants of mothers who smoke but also those exposed to cigarette smoke from partners who smoke or environments that cause exposure to smoke.

In another study, 505 pregnant women were assessed for prenatal exposure to pollution and the development of atopic disease in the first year of their infant's life. The prevalence of atopic dermatitis was significantly associated with prenatal exposure to PM10, nitrogen oxide compounds, and carbon monoxide. (93) In a separate urban birth cohort study performed in the United States, exposure to butyl benzyl phthalate from plastics during pregnancy was associated with early eczema development by two years of age. (94)

All these studies collectively suggest that outdoor air pollution is one of the potent risk factors for the development of atopic dermatitis. In addition to the effects on the prevalence of eczema, outdoor air pollution also influences the severity of skin symptoms in patients with atopic dermatitis. One study found that on days when eczema patients experienced worse symptoms, the concentrations of outdoor PM10, PM2.5, toluene, and total volatile organic compounds were higher, and vice versa; on days when they reported no deterioration in their symptoms, air pollution was seen to be lower. (95)

Another exposure that can significantly impact eczema but generally only occurs once or twice a year is that caused by fireworks. They release nitrogen dioxide, sulphur dioxide, carbon dioxide, and ozone. Eczema and asthma sufferers should ideally watch fireworks from inside to avoid breathing the polluted air. Highly sensitive people will also benefit from using an air filtration device at these times. Having efficient double glazing also reduces air pollutants entering the living accommodation through the gaps in the windows.

Air Pollution (Indoor)

The air we breathe inside our homes and workplaces can also cause problems with eczema. For example, in a German birth cohort study, redecorating activities, such as painting, laying new floor coverings, and purchasing brand-new furniture before birth and during the first year of life, were associated with the development of atopic dermatitis before the age of six years. (69) Another study conducted in Korea, involving 380 children below seven years of age, found similar results and showed an association between eczema severity and indoor home redecorating activities, such as painting, laying new floor coverings, and wallpapering. In fact, having a history of living in a newly built house during the first year of life was positively correlated with atopic dermatitis development in school children. (96) *Allergy, Asthma, and Immunology Research* published an article reporting that the formaldehyde used in building materials and many consumer products can exacerbate eczema symptoms and severity by over 79%, even when exposure is at much lower rates (13.6 ppb on average) than that declared by the World Health Organization to be considered safe (80 ppb). Formaldehyde is commonly found in chemical cleaning products, cosmetics, paints, and furniture. In addition, some common preservatives, such as Diazolidinyl urea and imidazolidinyl urea, trimethylolnitromethan, DMDM hydantoin, benzylhmiformal, and quaternium-15, are formaldehyde-based and can cause eczema flare-ups from both skin contact with the products and from breathing the formaldehyde fumes they release. Therefore, they should all be avoided by eczema sufferers.

Another case-control study comprising 198 eczema sufferers and 202 control subjects aged 3-8 years old found that eczema symptoms in children were associated with the concentration of butyl benzyl phthalate in dust collected from their bedrooms. Butyl benzyl phthalate is a plasticiser used in vinyl flooring, polyvinyl chloride (P.V.C.), and artificial leather. Although its use has declined since it was declared toxic by the European Chemical Bureau, it may still be present in these types of products. Unfortunately, butyl benzyl phthalate vapours are easily absorbed by the human body in various ways, including dermally (through the skin).

Other common indoor air pollutants come from furniture, air conditioning units, stoves, emulsion, construction materials, cloths, duvets, carpets, and even the human body itself. Toluene is known to increase eczema severity in direct correlation to increases in its pollution levels. Concerns about indoor air pollution became an even greater concern in 2020 and 2021, as in addition to spending most of our time inside, at home, school, or work, lockdowns prevented us from being able to travel between those places, increasing our exposure to indoor air pollution even more. Toluene is a common ingredient in adhesives, artificial fragrances (one of the reasons plug-in air fresheners can trigger eczema flare-ups), ink, nylon, plastic bottles, and tobacco smoke. It is also used to make benzene, which is particularly hazardous for eczema sufferers.

How does benzene affect eczema? Benzene and its metabolites, especially hydroquinone and benzoquinone, can influence the responses of mast cells and basophils together with other cells, such as helper T cells, macrophages, and monocytes. In a study performed on a group of 3-year-old children, exposure to benzene, ethylbenzene, and chlorobenzene was related to them having higher percentages of IL-4-producing helper T cells, which we have already seen are linked to favouring the development and persistence of atopic dermatitis. An increase of only 1 part per billion (which is minuscule) of benzene concentration in the blood was associated with a 27.38% increase in eczema symptoms. In addition, animal and human experimental models have shown an increase in the number of both inflammatory Th2 cytokines and IgE levels after exposure to air pollutants such as diesel exhaust fumes, nitrogen dioxide, and polycyclic aromatic hydrocarbons from petrol engines and tobacco. (98)

Another mechanism by which these chemicals affect eczema is by increasing water loss through the skin. Exposure to gaseous pollutants such as formaldehyde, nitrogen dioxide, and volatile organic compounds causes increased water evaporation from the skin in patients with atopic dermatitis. (100) In the case of volatile organic compounds, such as those from paints, varnish, and Danish tung oil for wooden countertops, the increased water loss could be seen in the skin after only 48 hours of exposure. (101) Many people are aware of volatile organic compounds in paints and solvents as they have seen the tins labelled with the volatile organic compound level, ranging from low to extremely high. However, volatile organic compounds are also present in detergents, degreasers, petrol, and natural gas. They can even be in nail varnishes and cosmetics. A source of formaldehyde that most people are unaware of is Teflon and non-stick cookware. When over-heated or damaged, they can release dangerous fumes, including formaldehyde, which in addition to being harmful to eczema sufferers, can also cause sickness with flu-like symptoms. This is common enough to have earned the nickname Teflon flu.

Many years after we had freed our children from the clutches of eczema, one daughter suddenly regressed and suffered eczema flare-ups again just days after we moved into a brand-new home, complete with its generous supply of formaldehyde fumes and other toxic by-products of the building and decorating processes. That experience prompted me to search for scientific documents relating to eczema and exposure to building and decorating toxins. Please be aware that brand new is not best when you are susceptible to eczema development unless you can insist that the building company use non-toxic paints and flooring in your unit. Even then, it would still be necessary to use an air filtration device to remove the toxins from the actual building process. Newly purchased modern furniture can also release toxic gases at elevated levels for the first three months, with some continuing to release these fumes for years!

Apart from taking care when decorating, using non-toxic paints (which you can purchase easily online), and making a conscious effort to buy natural over man-made furnishings and floorings, it is not always possible to control the amount of pollution in our environment, nor is it easy to pack up and move home. The best way to mitigate air pollution inside your home is to use HEPA air filtration systems with enough units to cover every room or to install a whole house system. You also need to avoid certain actions during peak traffic flow hours, such as outdoor exercise, opening windows, or, if the kids have eczema, allowing them to play outside during rush hours.

Dust mites are another frequent problem for eczema sufferers. Researchers have conducted skin prick tests on children with eczema and found that over 90% had elevated allergic responses to house dust mites. (117) Another interesting study published in the *European Journal of Allergy and Clinical Immunology* tested the effect of dust-mite removal in the environment of eczema patients. They separated patients into two groups and assessed them for six months: the control group used regular mattress covers and vacuum cleaners, and the test group used Gortex mattress covers, HEPA filter vacuum cleaners, and a household spray containing tannic acid and benzyl alcohol to kill dust mites. The researchers found, in their words, "highly significant benefits" in the skin of the eczema patients in the dust mite-limiting group, with "the biggest improvements seen in those who had the most severe eczema." (118). I urge caution, though, if you try to replicate this anti-dust-mite spray at home, as ewg.org lists benzyl alcohol as a potential allergen, with a higher risk factor when used as a spray that could be inhaled. Tannic acid is not listed as harmful by the Environmental Working Group. However, repeated use can cause the discolouration of light-coloured materials such as carpets.

Gortex mattress covers and a HEPA filter vacuum have no safety concerns.

A vast amount of literature confirms the link between dust mite allergy and eczema severity. However, it is questionable whether the allergy causes the original eczema or develops due to the defective skin barrier allowing penetration of the dust mite allergen to trigger a subsequent immune response and perpetuate eczema flares. Either way, it is clearly beneficial for eczema sufferers to reduce their exposure by adopting Gortex mattresses and pillow covers, vacuums with HEPA filters, and potentially using alcohol or tannin-based dust cleaning products.

Another toxin frequently shown in scientific literature to increase the prevalence of eczema is mould exposure. Studies conducted in China, Japan, Spain, and Finland have confirmed that exposure to mould during pregnancy increases the prevalence of eczema development in infants. Furthermore, children exposed to mould in the home also have an increased risk of developing eczema. (119,120,121,122) Mould appears to affect the differentiation of helper T cells, favouring the Th2 production and increasing the production of IL-5 and IL-13 inflammatory cytokines. (123) Mould exposure can also cause the release of thymic stromal lymphopoietin by keratinocyte cells and triggers the involvement of reactive oxygen species in the skin, causing eczema flare-ups. (124) We saw in Chapter 7 that thymic stromal lymphopoietin release kicks off the inflammatory cycle with the dendritic cells 'waking up' and releasing inflammatory cytokines to summon the immune cells to the skin. In addition to this, mould exposure can also cause mould sensitivity, resulting in an allergic response and histamine release on subsequent exposures. Interestingly, vitamin D3, which is often seen to be deficient in eczema sufferers, has been shown to moderate the Th2 response to mould exposure. (125)

Heavy Metals

Moving on to look at heavy metal exposure, a study in North Korea assessed whether there was any association between exposure to three heavy metals (lead, cadmium, and mercury) and the development of atopic diseases, namely asthma, atopic dermatitis, and allergic rhinitis. The study found that heavy metals directly activate Th2 cells, consequently increasing the production of Th2 inflammatory cytokines. Our immune cells are known to react to heavy metals as they are poisonous. This is called an adjuvant effect and is why toxic metals are often used in vaccines. By acting as an adjuvant to stimulate the immune response, they increase the sensitisation of the immune cells to the viral proteins in the vaccines. However, heavy metal toxicity also increases sensitisation to antigens and potential allergen proteins injected simultaneously in the vaccines, such as egg albumin (a protein in egg white), in which many vaccines are cultured. (There are growing concerns amongst some researchers that heavy metals in vaccines can also stimulate an immune response against human proteins from aborted fetal cells, which the adjuvants bind to in the vaccine. This may contribute to the development of infertility and auto-immune diseases by causing antibody production against our human cells.) The scientists in this North Korean study confirmed that having an overly dominant Th2 balance driven by elevated levels of heavy metals leads to a dysregulated immune system, causing other atopic conditions to develop via the thymic stromal lymphopoietin pathway that we covered in Chapter 7. In conclusion, the study positively associated all three metals with developing different atopic conditions. They found that having elevated lead levels in the bloodstream was associated with the development of asthma, atopic dermatitis, and the Allergic March, whereas elevated blood levels of cadmium were related to the development of both asthma and allergic rhinitis but not eczema. All three tested heavy metals (lead, mercury, and cadmium) were shown to be associated with airflow obstruction in Korean adults. (69)

The elephant in the room we are not supposed to talk about for fear of being labelled anti-vaxxers is that of heavy metal contamination in vaccines. Researchers have been raising the alarm over this topic for decades. Still, Big Pharma and the medical establishment refuse to acknowledge the elephant and indeed seem to actively discredit anyone trying to point it out.

Back in 1992, an excellent study showed a clear link between the aluminium-based D.T.P. vaccine (diphtheria, typhoid, and polio) and the development of eczema related to aluminium allergy. The scientists stated that aluminium allergy is positively associated with an increased risk of developing atopic dermatitis. The risk is even greater if the pneumococcal vaccine is given at the same time (which it usually is now). They recommended that aluminium allergy tests be performed if a child develops eczema after immunisation, especially as subsequent vaccine doses will also contain aluminium, potentially triggering an even more severe allergic reaction and increased severity of eczema. Another study published in 2016 confirmed these findings and examined whether delaying vaccines would influence the risk of developing eczema. They concluded that delaying infant vaccinations until after one year of age directly correlated with a reduced risk of developing atopic dermatitis. (18) The scientists conducting this study were not anti-vaxxers but instead highlighted the need to consider the impact of injecting these metals into children at ever-increasing doses. It is shameful that this valuable and insightful research has not been disseminated to family practitioners. Most are blissfully ignorant of the risks inherent in following the vaccine schedules. They still believe and spout the false narrative that there is no link between eczema development and the vaccination of babies. Consequently, babies are still not tested for aluminium allergy or aluminium toxicity when they develop eczema after immunisations. It is equally shameful that parents are not given these facts and the option of delaying vaccines, especially in families that are already known to be at risk for atopic diseases.

A further issue with aluminium, apart from allergy, is that it detrimentally impacts the ability to produce a healthy skin barrier. The *American Journal of Dermatology* published a study in September 2019 showing that mice skin models contaminated with aluminium experienced disruption in the processing of profilaggrin to filaggrin, and the mice developed eczema rashes as a result. Their study indicated that the presence of aluminium in the skin caused the early death of skin cells before they had been filled sufficiently with keratin protein and before the completion of profilaggrin to filaggrin processing. (18) This would directly reduce the amount of keratin, histidine, and other S100 proteins that should have filled the keratinocyte cells, resulting in a reduced level of natural moisturising factor and impairing the integrity of the skin barrier. (Well, that sounds just like eczema to me.) I do NOT believe it is a coincidence that infant eczema usually appears at eight weeks of age, which is the exact same time infant vaccines are given. Both my first two children were very sick after their 8-week baby vaccines, and 48 hours later, they developed eczema. My doctor refused to accept that there was any link between eczema and the vaccines and even went as far as to tell me that it had been studied and proven to be nothing more than coincidental. I do not know where he got his studies, but a simple search on google scholar reveals quite the contrary. With my subsequent children, I had not yet studied this issue for myself and still believed vaccines were necessary to protect my children. However, my concerns about eczema development prompted me to test my theory that these shots were causing eczema in my children. Therefore, I delayed their first injections as long as I could. My third and fourth children had no vaccines until they were 5 and 6 months old, respectively, and they remained very healthy despite the practice nurse and doctor repeatedly telling me I was putting them in danger the whole time. When I eventually gave them their first vaccinations, like clockwork, they both developed eczema 48 hours later. Their doctor still maintains it is just coincidental.

The country that has consistently shown the lowest rates of eczema across all age ranges is Japan. (19) In addition to having one of the highest consumptions of fermented foods, they also have one of the lowest rates of infant vaccinations and consequent aluminium exposure. Is this just another coincidence? Personally, I do not think so.

A doctor in Oregon in the United States conducted a study on his patients to assess the long-term health impacts of vaccination on children. His practice consisted of roughly half vaccinated children and half non-vaccinated, so he was in an excellent position to do such an analysis. His results were shocking. His pediatric appointments for ear infections, throat infections, conjunctivitis, eczema, asthma, attention deficit hyperactivity disorder, and autism were almost exclusively for vaccinated children; he only rarely had appointments booked for health issues with unvaccinated children. His tests on aluminium levels in vaccinated children who followed the United States vaccination schedule found that their blood levels of aluminium far exceeded the safety levels even for adults in the first 2.5 years of their lives. This study should have rung alarm bells and prompted further investigation, but when it was published, he was hauled before the medical board and threatened with being struck off the medical register as he was a 'threat to public health'. His study was retracted, despite him never retracting it himself and having none of his study information disputed or proven false. Do you remember the billion-dollar question I shared at the beginning of the book? "Would it make good business sense to manufacture a product that actually cures eczema?" Bearing in mind that vaccine manufacturers are immune from all liability for injury or harm that results from anyone taking vaccines and that the same companies making the vaccines also produce profitable products to treat any side effects they cause, perhaps we should also be asking what the real purpose of vaccines is. Is the vaccine agenda really to improve our children's health? Who do you think benefits most from them, our children or the pharmaceutical company's profit margins? In addition, the narrative that vaccines caused the eradication of many diseases, such as measles, is entirely false. Careful research of the historical data of these diseases shows that they were almost eradicated by improved sanitation and nutrition before the vaccines were ever bought to market. However, using cleverly enlarged excerpts of selected portions of disease data charts, the public (and medical trainees) can easily be fooled into believing the improvements were bought about solely by the vaccines.

There are other common sources of aluminium exposure that eczema patients need to be aware of, both to avoid increased exposure impacting the skin barrier function and because you or your child could have developed an allergy to aluminium. It is commonly added to cosmetics such as eyeshadows, foundations, and blushers as it contributes a shiny or illuminating effect to the products. Many deodorants and antiperspirants also contain aluminium and have been linked to the development of breast cancer. Aluminium cooking pans, trays, and foil are other common sources of aluminium toxicity. When food is heated in aluminium, especially if it has a high fat or high water content, it can become contaminated. Tetra Pak cartons for liquid storage are lined with aluminium and can be another source of exposure. According to Christopher Exley, PhD, aluminium is particularly dangerous in the form of Al3+(aq), which is the form that is found in water. Exley states that they know unequivocally that it is biologically reactive in that form and will bind to other molecules, rendering them ineffective. Imagine the aluminium binding to the water molecules in your blood, preventing them from being able to attach to the essential metal ions such as magnesium. (116) This has enormous health implications.

Aluminium exposure has been implicated in many disease states, including neurodegenerative diseases such as Alzheimer's. This is not surprising, considering it is present in the annual flu vaccines given to the elderly. However, considering the severe consequences of aluminium exposure on skin processing, this alone should be reason enough for eczema patients to exercise even greater diligence and to source personal care and cookware products that do not contain aluminium. All forms of aluminium can break down in the right conditions to release the toxic Al3+(aq). (116) Clearly, the safety of injecting aluminium directly into the bloodstream, which is itself an aqueous solution full of biomolecules, should be allowed to be questioned, for the sake of our children at the very least, but also for the sake of our elderly relatives who seem to be developing neurological degeneration at increasing rates, after a lifetime of vaccines, and particularly annual flu shots in their later years. As a side note, Exley and his team have examined many donated brains from deceased people and, without fail, found that those with low levels of aluminium had not developed Alzheimer's, Parkinson's, multiple sclerosis, or autism. In contrast, those with high levels of aluminium had indeed developed these diseases. Aluminium travels in the body and can persist in tissues for decades, which enables toxicity to build over time. Consider Exley's research in combination with the findings of the doctor I mentioned in Oregon. Is it any wonder that so many children are suffering from autism, attention deficit hyperactivity disorder, and learning difficulties if the aluminium in their vaccines is taking them over the adult safety levels and persisting in their brain tissue for decades? Or is that just another elephant in the room, like the involvement of vaccines in the development of eczema? Interestingly, because the gut microbiome has such a vital role in breaking down heavy metals and other toxins, you can see why those infants who have inherited a deficient microbiome either from a C-section birth, by the mother being given antibiotics whilst in labour, or by not being breastfed, all have an increased risk of vaccine damage. (37)

Apart from aluminium, nickel, cobalt, and chromium are considered the most common metals causing the contact dermatitis form of eczema. However, other metals can also cause hypersensitivity reactions, such as cadmium, lead, platinum, mercury, and copper. If someone has experienced chronic internal exposure, they can become sensitised to external exposure. You may wonder how we can have internal exposure, but several studies have suggested that metal implants used for various medical purposes, such as intravascular stents, dental implants, cardiac pacemakers, or implanted gynecologic devices, can be sources of sensitisation. All these metals have been shown to increase both allergic tendencies and inflammatory responses in the body. The most common sources of mercury contamination are amalgam fillings in teeth, additives in drugs and vaccines, or eating entrails and mercury-contaminated seafood. Mercury is known to bind to the epithelial cells of the gastrointestinal tract and the skin, as well as to the hair, thyroid gland, liver, pancreas, kidneys, and brain. Mercury contamination also interferes with the effective manufacture of S100 skin proteins and hinders our detox ability. (69) It also suppresses the action of the microbes in the gut that would keep yeast colonies, such as candida, under control. Thus mercury contamination can be a cause of repeated yeast infections. If you have old amalgam fillings that contain mercury, consider taking a test for mercury contamination, as these fillings can deteriorate over time and leach mercury into the surrounding tissues. I have experienced this personally after cracking two teeth containing old amalgam fillings. As a result of the repeated and particularly nasty candida-infected rashes that ensued, I opted to have all the mercury fillings removed from my mouth and replaced with bio-compatible materials. I have not had any yeast infections since.

Contact dermatitis-type eczema can also be caused by other chemical additives and preservatives used in cosmetics, fragrances, hair dyes, perming lotions, nail polishes, etc. Ingredients such as balsam of Peru, cinnamic aldehyde, parabens, formaldehyde, and formaldehyde releasers, including iodopropynyl butylcarbamate, methyldibromo glutaronitrile, and paraphenylenediamine have all been identified as causing contact dermatitis type rashes. (69) Isothiazolinones (including methylisothiazolinone and methylchloroisothiazolinone, commonly listed as simply M.I. or M.C.I. on ingredient lists) are preservatives used in liquid products to prevent bacteria from multiplying, which you need to be particularly careful of. They are found in a vast array of products, including shampoos and hair care items, moisturisers, cosmetics, detergents and laundry care products, carpet glues and adhesives, paints and solvents, and sunscreen lotions. They seem to be working their way into everything. However, allergies to these chemicals have increased at an alarming rate, which has now been recognised as a global problem, resulting in the United Nations declaring them to be strong allergens. The contact dermatitis rash that results from the allergic reactions to these chemicals can be pretty severe and can affect anywhere on the body or scalp, even in areas where you have not used any products containing them. Allergy tests can be performed by a patch test, but the test gives false negative results in around 60% of cases. This is because many clinics only test for allergy to methylisothiazolinone, whereas most people react to methylisothiazolinone and methylchloroisothiazolinone combined. They do frequently occur in combination in products. It can be hard to detect the source of methylisothiazolinone and methylchloroisothiazolinone, particularly if they are released as fumes from adhesives or paints containing these chemicals. Still, if you have been renovating, purchasing an air purification device is advisable to remove these airborn triggers. (110)

Remember when I advised you previously to check the ingredients of the products you use; if they contain words so long you struggle to pronounce the names, then most likely they are not healthy for you. Please check the Environmental Working Group website to find brands and products that are non-toxic and start transitioning to clean personal care to limit exposure to toxic soup ingredients.

Lead is another toxic metal that has been implicated in eczema development. In one study, researchers checked and recorded the blood samples of women in their last trimester for lead. Their infants were observed after birth, and their eczema development was recorded and compared to the pre-term lead levels in the mother's blood. It was found that maternal blood lead concentration in late pregnancy was positively associated with a higher risk of these infants developing atopic dermatitis by six months of age, especially in baby boys. (70) A common source of lead exposure is deteriorating lead pipes in older homes. In America, the use of lead pipes was not banned until 1986 and much later in the United Kingdom. However, that applied to new-build homes, so any homes built before this are still likely to have mains water supplied through lead pipes. You can replace them at an exorbitant cost, but even then, installing a whole-house water filter is still advisable, as lead is only one of many contaminants to be found in our water.

Food Additives

Besides food, several chemical substances added to food to improve its properties are associated with non-allergic food sensitivities. Food additives can be added to food at any stage of production, processing, treatment, packaging, transportation, or storage. Various food preservatives (parabens, benzoates, citric acid, nitrates and nitrites, sorbic acid, sulphating agents), antioxidants such as butylated hydroxyanisole and butylated hydroxytoluene (listed as BHT), artificial dyes (tartrazine, erythrosine, sunset yellow, brilliant black, plus anything called FD&C colours), stabilisers (EDTA, carrageenan, guar gum), flavourings, and taste enhancers (monosodium glutamate, disodium-5 ribonucleotide), emulsifiers (Arabic gum, karaya gum, lecithin, propylene glycol), and artificial sweeteners (aspartame, acesulfame K, saccharin) have all been studied to see if they cause hypersensitivity reactions. Although the prevalence of reactions to their use in food is typically very low in the general population, it was increased in people with eczema. Aspartame can be particularly problematic for eczema sufferers as it converts to formaldehyde as it breaks down in the body. Individual reactivity to food additives varies. Not everyone will react to the same ones, even if they all have eczema. (69) Therefore, it is important to be aware of the possibility of food additive reactions and to keep a food tracker to assess them. Below is a list of some common food additives and the health implication that have been associated with them. After reading them, you will see why I advise eating a natural, unprocessed diet. Unfortunately, the more food companies play with our foods; the more corrupt they are likely to be.

E621 MSG (flavour enhancer) can cause skin rashes, hyperactivity, chest pain, headaches, nausea, and asthma attacks.

E635/E627/E631 (flavour enhancers) can cause rash, allergies, and anaphylaxis.

E102 tartrazine (Orange colour) causes hyperactivity and asthma. Many packages containing it now carry warnings about its effect on children's behaviour.

E512 (colour) can cause vomiting, diarrhoea, and headaches.

E951 aspartame (a very common artificial sweetener) can cause headaches, seizures, and mood and memory problems. Additionally, it converts to formaldehyde in the body.

E210/213 (preservative) can affect digestion and trigger allergies.

E320 (preservative) can cause hyperactivity, and some articles link it to cancer development.

E226 (preservative) can cause breathing problems, low blood pressure, and anaphylaxis.

E220 (preservative) can lead to bronchial problems and anaphylaxis.

E124 (Ponceau 4: has over 100 different names) causes hyperactivity and attention deficit hyperactivity disorder-type behaviour.

E151 (black food colour) can trigger asthma attacks and allergies.

E129 (red food colour) causes asthma and rhinitis.

Although they are not food additives, some plants contain toxins called oxalates and solanine that can affect eczema when you handle them rather than eat them; thus, it is essential to mention these. Anyone with hand eczema needs to be rather careful of vegetables containing oxalates and solanines, as they can cause extreme itching and inflammation after peeling the skins or cutting them. Plants such as eddoes, dasheen roots, and dasheen leaves are particularly potent hand irritants. Some people also break out in contact dermatitis when they handle garlic, onions, nightshade plants (tomatoes, potatoes, eggplant, peppers, chillies, etc.), spinach, and citrus. It is not always apparent that you are reacting to these foods, as the itching and inflammation can start many hours after you peel them. I experienced this myself after peeling eddoes whilst living in Trinidad. Still, because of the delayed reaction (I would wake up in the middle of the night with bright red, intensely itching palms and fingers), it was months before I realised that peeling eddoes was causing it. If you cook with these foods, you can minimise the risk of reactions by either wearing gloves or coating your hands in olive oil before handling them. I prefer to wear gloves as I don't particularly appreciate having slippery hands when holding sharp knives.

There are other unlisted contaminants in foods, such as nickel, which can be found in beans, coffee, soy, chocolate, lentils, shellfish, and spinach, along with mould and mycotoxins commonly found in dried foods. Therefore, reactions to these foods may not be caused by the foods themselves but to the mould or nickel. If so, changing to an uncontaminated brand may resolve the problem with that food item.

Plastics

I have already spoken about the toxicity of bisphenol A, butyl benzyl phthalate (BBP), and benzene in plastics. They are such prevalent pollutants that it is worth mentioning them again and re-iterating my advice to transition away from all synthetic furnishings, plastic storage containers, plastic drinking water bottles, plastic cling wrap, and plastic or polystyrene food containers. Plastic residues can build up in our cells and have even been found in the placentas of newborn infants. It is horrifying that we are now so toxically overloaded that we are passing chemicals on to our children in the womb. It is a toxic burden that neither we, our children, nor our environment need.

Pesticides

It is still commonly believed in many countries that Roundup is among the safest pesticides. This idea is still spread by manufacturers, mostly in the reviews they promote, often cited in toxicological evaluations of glyphosate-based herbicides. Here in the Caribbean, the "Roundup is safe" narrative is still believed. Consequently, Roundup™ is sprayed liberally almost everywhere, destroying the vitally important bee and monarch butterfly populations required for pollinating plants and also decimating the microbiomes of the human inhabitants who eat the sprayed produce. Researchers found the chemical cocktail in Round-up™ 125 times more toxic than glyphosate alone. Moreover, despite its reputation, Roundup was by far the most toxic among the tested herbicides and insecticides. The vast differences between published industry rhetoric and scientific data can most likely be attributed to huge economic interests, which have been found to falsify health risk assessments and prioritise profits over people. (73) I have seen graphs plotting the rates of food allergy diagnosis and specific cancer diagnoses with the rates of glyphosate use in agricultural farming. The graphs are almost perfectly correlated.

I wrote previously about the dangers of pesticides. The same bacterial pathways targeted by them are also used by the friendly microbes in our gut. When we eat pesticide-laden foods, we destroy our inner rainforest and trigger a tsunami of health implications, which may not even become apparent for many years. To maintain our health or to regain it, we must eat clean, organic produce. The more we purchase it, the more we create demand, and the more profitable it becomes to produce. The only way we can genuinely influence agriculture practices is by wielding the power of our wallet. Buy organic or grow your own.

I have heard of some people washing their fruits and vegetables in dishwashing liquid to scrub off pesticide residues. Unfortunately, this is just replacing one chemical cocktail with another, as exposure to cinnamaldehyde and other ingredients in dishwashing detergents has also been shown to decrease the butyrate production by the gut microbes, detrimentally affecting their ability to produce branch chain fatty acids. If you cannot source organic produce, the most effective way to clean your plant foods is to soak them in an aluminium-free sodium bicarbonate solution for 15 minutes and lightly rub the skins to remove the residues. (102) It will not remove everything though, just external residues; some of the pesticides would have soaked into the soil and been absorbed into the food via the root system.

Other Toxins

Mould and mycotoxins are other culprits that can cause or exacerbate eczema. In 2016, researchers wrote of a woman who had a persistent eczema rash and had been taking approximately six courses of antibiotics and steroids annually for the previous 15 years. The researchers tested her home for mould contamination and found it was indeed contaminated, the predominant strain being *Aspergillus*. The patient was also tested for mould allergy, and when she tested positive, she moved out of her home. Only two weeks after leaving, her rash had resolved. This lady had suffered for 15 years, repeatedly being prescribed steroids and antibiotics, which brought a host of side effects along with their supposed treatment. Instead, all she needed to do was move out of her mould-infested home. (115) Do not underestimate the consequences of mould exposure. Clinicalposters.com lists 73 known health implications of mould exposure, and that number does not even include the effects of mould allergy. Mould can develop in basements, inadequately ventilated areas such as bedrooms, loft spaces, kitchens, bathrooms, and any areas that have experienced water damage or flooding, especially basements. It can also occur in air conditioning units that have not been cleaned adequately or efficiently and old water filters that have been left installed but not maintained or replaced. Black mould is particularly hazardous, but any mould exposure can cause serious health implications. Tests can ascertain if you have toxicity issues from mould contamination, but you may need to approach an integrative or functional medical professional to obtain these. They will also be able to assist you with specific detox protocols for the type of exposure you have experienced. Please be aware that if mould is a problem in your home, the best solution may be to move out entirely and live somewhere else that is mould free. Yes, it would be disruptive and expensive, but if mould is the reason you have eczema, you could be facing the same circumstances as the lady in the research study; 15 years of ineffective medication compared to complete healing in 2 weeks by moving out. I know which one I would choose.

Parasites

Some forms of eczema are caused or exacerbated by parasitic infections in the gut or the skin. Following the protocols in this book will provide a generally more inhospitable environment for pathogens and parasites. This is often enough to eliminate eczema.

As mentioned previously, parasite infections have been shown to cause an increased allergic nature, higher circulating IgE levels and increased serum levels of histamine and other granular mediators from degranulating immune cells. I believe this is because your body 'expects' any invasions entering via the skin and the gut lining to be parasites and is therefore using the immune arsenal designed for parasite infections against undigested protein particles, whether they be from food or environmental sources. If, after working through these chapters, you still have a problem with eczema flare-ups, then you should contact an integrative or functional medical professional to request tests to ascertain if you require specialised treatment for specific pathogens, parasites, toxins, or nutritional deficiencies.

Detoxing Action Points

Many detox procedures are the same regardless of the type of toxicity, but there are also specific protocols that are helpful for particular toxin exposures.

1. **Remove the exposure.** The first thing to do when detoxing is to either remove yourself from the exposure to the toxin or remove the toxin from exposing you. When it comes to looking after your health, both you and toxins cannot exist in the same place. There is simply no point in trying to detox if the source of the poison is still contaminating you. Eat organic, unprocessed foods and limit your intake of mercury-contaminated fish. Switch to natural, non-toxic personal care and cleaning products. Throw out your aluminium cooking foil and replace your aluminium cookware with stainless steel or cast-iron ceramic-coated pans. I recently read about some tests on cookware to assess for toxins, which found Le Creuset to be the safest cookware, which I was happy about because this is my favourite cookware brand. It is a higher premium but lasts far longer. As with anything in life, you typically get what you pay for.

    In summary, do not allow people to smoke in your home, move home if necessary to remove yourself from indoor pollution such as mould, formaldehyde, butyl benzyl phthalate, traffic pollution, etc., and consider investing in a HEPA air filtration device to remove airborne allergens and toxins. In addition, use Gortex dust mite covers and natural alcohol sprays to kill dust mites.

2. **Exercise.** When we exercise, we increase our heart rate, breathe faster, increase our oxygen intake, and increase the speed at which our blood circulates, carrying nutrients and oxygen to

our cells and waste products away from them. We also sweat more as our body temperature increases; sweating is an excellent detox mechanism. Some eczema patients experience flare-ups when sweating; however, this can be caused by petroleum-based emollients blocking the pores and causing the sweat to leach out into the surrounding tissues, leading to an allergic response developing against your own sweat. In this case, use a fan whilst exercising, and ensure you shower and moisturise immediately afterwards. Make sure you use natural moisturisers that allow the sweat to exit via the pores. Drinking homemade high-dose vitamin C drinks will also lower your histamine levels and allergic response whilst exercising. Saunas are also helpful for increasing circulation and sweating; the same advice applies to reduce the risk of skin irritation.

3. **Regular bowel movements.** We all need to take our trash out every day. Otherwise, our houses will become polluted with bad smells, toxic food remains, and undesirable pathogens. Our body is no different in that respect. It is imperative to excrete waste at least once a day. Eating a diet rich in vegetables and legumes/pulses (if you can tolerate them) will aid in speeding the transition time of waste through the gut. Coffee is a natural laxative, and if you are not sensitive to caffeine, it is a helpful aid to bowel regularity as it increases gallbladder contractions. TUDCA supplements are another useful remedy. Constipation is the enemy of detoxification as the longer your waste sits inside you, the more it deteriorates, increasing its toxic and unfavourable bacterial load and, in addition, increasing your histamine burden. You also continue to absorb water from your stools for as long as they are inside you. Thus, as the toxicity of your stool increases, so does the rancidity of the water you are absorbing. Diversifying the plants in your diet will also help you improve your gut microbiome diversity. This widening of the variety of gut microbes will help your body break down and eliminate toxins in the gut. Remember the advice to eat rainbows and try to incorporate a new plant food every week. A valuable cleansing aid is taking either organic coffee or saltwater enemas

twice a week for two weeks. These involve using an enema bag to insert the warm liquid into the rectum and then holding it inside for as long as possible. They are very effective at clearing old waste and parasites from the colon. It is not usually easy to hold the fluid inside, but in the case of coffee, it increases bile production in the liver and stimulates the bowel to excrete more waste. Holding onto the coffee as tightly as you can for as long as possible also activates the Vagus nerve, lowering stress levels and improving gut health.

Interestingly, coffee enemas have been used for medical purposes for many years. They were used in World War 1 as effective pain relief when anaesthetics were in short supply. They have been shown to assist in lowering the burden of toxic waste metabolites and increasing beneficial compounds such as Glutathione S-Transferase, which has a major role in clearing free radicals. They are also an integral part of many natural cancer healing protocols. Holistic health clinics can assist you with these enemas, or you can purchase the enema kits online to D.I.Y. the procedure at home. When using any form of enema, it is crucial to ensure you are replenishing the friendly microbes by eating a diet that supports good microbial health and either eating anaerobic ferments or taking high-spectrum probiotics.

4. **Sleep.** The next protocol is to ensure adequate and good-quality sleep. Our brain cells, as well as our bodies, detox while we sleep. We also conduct much of our healing processes while we sleep. For this reason, work to establish excellent sleep routines, restore your circadian rhythm, and ensure your bedroom is dark for maximum melatonin production. Refer to the previous chapter for guidelines on how to reduce sleep stress.

5. **Vitamin C.** Ascorbates from vitamin C bind to lead and help carry it from the body. They also counteract free-radical damage, lower histamine levels, and help to increase bowel movements, which will aid in expelling toxins from the body faster. I have spoken of vitamin C quite extensively in this book, and I re-iterate its importance in your eczema healing journey.

6. **Water.** Water can either be a source of poisoning or an aid to detoxing, depending on the quality of your water. I advise getting your water supply tested for contaminants and fitting a whole house filter with a drinking water filter if funds permit. Although I do not like drinking from plastic water bottles, there are two brands of bottled water that have been studied and PROVEN to help detox aluminium from the body. Although the research was conducted by scientists looking to reduce aluminium exposure in Alzheimer's patients, it is very valuable information for eczema patients too, due to the deleterious effects of aluminium on the skin barrier function. These brands of water are Acilis and Volvic. Their benefit is derived from the high silica content in the natural springs they are bottled from. Natural silica binds to aluminium and carries it out of the body in the urine. (116) Fiji water is another brand that contains silica from a natural spring, but it was not included in the study. The researchers recommend drinking 1.5 litres of silica water daily to reduce the aluminium burden. Interestingly, Acilis water was named such because it is silica spelt backwards.

7. **Detox baths.** Detox baths and ionic footbaths can also be helpful to aid detoxing. With the use of footbaths, the water changes colour as the toxins are absorbed from the body; the detox effects continue for days afterwards as the ionic charge increases the ability of the cells to continue detoxing. Researchers found the heavy metal content in urine peaked three days after having an ionic foot detox bath. For this reason, I advise combining ionic footbaths with other detox methods for at least the next five days. Protocols such as drinking silica water, taking mineral supplements such as zinc, adding more green vegetables and herbal teas or tinctures to your diet, and taking a high-quality zeolite remedy to bind to the heavy metals and carry them from your body work very well together. People have used Epsom salt baths, Fulvic, diatomaceous earth, and chlorine dioxide successfully in their detox regimes. There are many others. If you wish to utilise these additional detox methods, do your research and seek professional advice so that you can detox under the care

of someone who can inform you of the correct dosage and any potential side effects.

8. **Nutrition.** Mineral deficiencies contribute to increased toxicity as minerals can bind to or chelate heavy metals. I covered this before in the chapter on nutrition. The electrolyte minerals potassium, calcium, and sodium all assist in the detox mechanisms, as does zinc. An excellent source of electrolytes is natural coconut water from green coconuts. Its electrolyte composition is said to be similar to that of human blood; indeed, it has even been used in place of blood transfusions when blood was unavailable.

Green plants are excellent detox aids as they contain chlorophyll and many nutrients that bind to and help excrete toxins. We should eat copious amounts of organic greens for optimal health. We can add them to salads, stews, soups, juices, smoothies, and teas. Cilantro is known to be excellent for its detoxing properties without any nasty side effects, as are the humble and often maligned dandelion and celery plants. Many are oblivious to the amazing healing benefits of the dandelion, viewing those bright yellow flowers and candy ball fluffs as annoying weeds that mar their lawns. However, every part of the dandelion is helpful for health; the roots, leaves, and flowers. Celery, on the other hand, is often avoided by people who simply dislike the taste. However, it is easy to disguise in smoothies and juices.

The blue-green algae chlorella helps to flush toxins out of the body. Ensure you purchase chlorella grown in clean waters, so it does not contain contaminants. Many more wonderful healing plants can be utilised to help with detoxing.

Apples contain malic acid, which can be another helpful aid to bind to and flush aluminium out of the body. When cooked with their skins, they contain valuable amounts of pectin, which helps to heal the gut lining and, in turn, helps to reduce the level of toxins leaching into the surrounding tissue and causing inflammation. Just ensure you buy organic, non-genetically modified apples, as otherwise, you will likely be consuming copious amounts of pesticides along with them.

Toxins complete the final strands of the spider web. You have learnt how toxins affect your microbiome, cellular health, absorption of nutrients, gene expression, skin barrier function, immune health, allergic sensitivities, and even your stress levels. So even though we now have a complete eczema spider web, with you trapped in the middle, we have been learning how to unravel these strands as we have progressed through this book.

If you are aiming to eat ten portions of fruit and vegetables a day in as many rainbow colours as possible, you will be providing your body with an abundance of nutrients and fibre to help you nourish your body and detox from pollutants. If you have been implementing the action points in all of the previous chapters, your detox pathways will be open, your toxin exposure minimised, your dietary deficiencies corrected, your healing mechanisms rebooted as you lower your stress levels, your sleep patterns restored, your allergen and pathogen exposure reduced, and your skin barrier function much improved. Consequently, you should now be seeing a significant improvement in your skin.

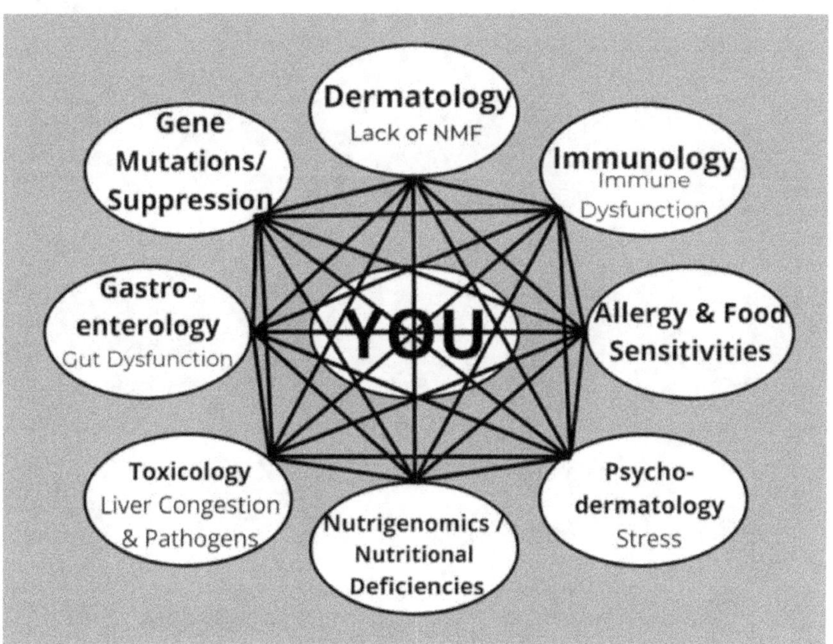

In the unlikely event that eczema flare-ups STILL plague you, despite actioning all the information in this book, then I highly recommend reaching out to me for 1:1 coaching or to a functional or integrative medical professional who can organise specific tests to ascertain if there are deeper issues to resolve, such as malabsorption, continuing nutritional deficiencies, parasites, or chronic infections. However, I have yet to see anyone who actions these protocols still having issues with their skin.

I congratulate you on reaching this stage of the book, and I commend your determination to learn and take action. I pray you have been greatly helped and have learnt much about eczema healing and the general protection of your health.

Now we can turn our attention to answering another question I am frequently asked: "Is there anything I can do to lower the risk of my children inheriting eczema?" Yes, there is, which is the topic of the next chapter.

SECTION 3:

ESCAPING THE WEB

13

Breaking the Chains

One of the concerns I frequently hear from eczema sufferers is that they are worried their future children will inherit it. Having suffered the torment themselves, they are understandably loathed to inflict that on their future offspring. However, it is important to realise that although there is a genetic component to eczema development, carrying these genes does NOT confer a certainty of suffering from it. In Chapter 6, I spoke of the genetic links and explained that our diet and lifestyle can largely influence disease genes through epigenetics. So, by changing your lifestyle and adopting healthy habits, especially concerning your food choices and avoiding toxins, you will go a long way to reducing the risk of your children developing eczema.

Within raw plant foods are biomolecules called microRNAs, which survive the digestive process. They act as silencers to the messenger RNAs that trigger the disease. This means that although your DNA may contain the code or gene mutation for a particular disease development, the microRNAs can silence the messenger molecules carrying out the code's instructions, thus turning it off. (22) As these silencer molecules can reside permanently within our germ cells (sperm and eggs), they can alter the genetic expression not just for us but also for our future generations.

In addition to actioning the education in this book to change your epigenetic factors, here are some additional helpful actions you can take (or avoid) that can stack the odds against your children developing eczema. First, seek to implement the five R's *before you conceive*. Remove, Restrict, Restore, Resist, and Refine.

BEFORE CONCEPTION (or as soon as possible after finding out you are pregnant)

1. Remove

Firstly, remove toxins from your environment. For example, do not eat fish with high levels of mercury, such as tuna and shark. Replace any cookware that is contaminating your food, such as aluminium-based pans and buy make-up and toiletries that are non-toxic and, in particular, aluminium-free.

Check yourself and your partner for toxic contamination to lead, mercury, and aluminium, and work to detox them before you attempt conception. Lead and mercury have been found in the placentas and increase the risk of eczema development. Aluminium interferes with the skin barrier function.

Move away from high traffic/high pollution areas. Living more than 50 meters away from main roads has been proven to lower the risk of children developing eczema and atopic diseases. (Although I would also be careful of living too near farmland in rural areas in case the crops are sprayed with pesticides and herbicides.) However, suppose it is not possible to move away. In that case, it is imperative to purchase air filtration devices for the home and to avoid being outside or opening the windows at times when pollution levels will be highest, such as rush hour.

In addition, ensure you filter your drinking water and use either a whole-house filter or, at the least, a chlorine filter for bathing.

2. Restrict

It is a good idea to get tested for IgA and IgG allergies, as antibodies can be passed on in breast milk and 'teach' the infant's immune system to see these foods as allergens. Once you identify your own food sensitivities, restrict your diet of these foods. Although it is sometimes easy to compromise with food intolerances as the reactions are not immediate, and we can feel like the pleasure of tasting those foods is worth the consequences, when you are considering conception, it is much better to avoid them entirely and allow the antibodies to those foods to minimise to protect your unborn child.

3. Restore

Get tested for, and treat, any nutritional deficiencies and work to restore a healthy and diverse gut microbiome by eating a wide variety of plant foods. Remember that the diversity of your gut microbiome directly reflects the diversity of the plant foods in your diet.

Take probiotics, particularly those containing the *Bifidobacterium, Lactobacillus Rhamnosous,* and *Acidophilus* strains, which have been shown to reduce the risk of eczema development.

Take clean omega-3 supplements, high-quality prenatal supplements, and a vitamin K supplement to help provide your baby with sufficient K for adequate blood clotting.

4. Resist

Resist buying or renting a brand-new home. They look lovely but come with a much higher burden of toxicity from the building and decorating materials. It is better to purchase or rent a home that is a few years old so that the levels of formaldehyde, butyl benzyl phthalate, toluene, and other contaminants have reduced significantly. Furthermore, be mindful of the nesting instinct that would have you decorating the house and nursery before your baby arrives. Any necessary refurbishments must be done with non-toxic, eco-friendly paints and furnishings. Check the ewg.org website for information on sources of clean supplies. Be careful of stripping paint in old houses as the previous layers may contain lead, which will cause you to be exposed if it is stripped or sanded. Consider if it is necessary to purchase brand-new furnishings. High-quality used furniture will reduce your exposure to off-gassing and will likely be much cheaper, helping your funds stretch further. Do NOT decorate before conception, while pregnant, or with a newborn. If decorating is necessary, vacate until it is completed and then use air filtration to clean the air of any dust and chemical residues.

5. Refine.

Refine your environment to create a space free from exposure to pollution, particularly from chemical cleaning and cosmetic products. Again, check out the ewg.org website for non-toxic brands.

By following these five Rs and learning to change your lifestyle to minimise your own disease risk, you are automatically laying a much better foundation for having healthy children.

DURING LABOR

In addition to these Rs, remember the research that shows vaginal birth and exclusive breastfeeding lowers the risk of developing atopic diseases of all types. If a C-section is necessary, ask about having the baby swabbed with the fluid from your birth canal to provide your baby with a healthy skin microbiome. Be careful of accepting intravenous antibiotics during labour, which will decimate the microbiome your baby should pick up on the way out. Ask for testing to prove that an infection exists and that it is a danger to your baby.

AFTER THE BIRTH

If you had a C-section, have antibiotic exposure, or are unable to breastfeed, supplement your baby with infant probiotics dissolved in filtered, boiled, and cooled water, as this has been shown to help manipulate their gut microbiome away from atopic tendencies.

Do your research before consenting to vitamin K injections for your newborn. Studies have shown the baby is similarly protected against excess bleeding by the mother taking supplemental vitamin K whilst pregnant and giving oral baby supplements. These, in my opinion, are safer than the shots. Vitamin K shots contain nasty ingredients such as polyethylene glycol and benzyl alcohol which can trigger allergic responses to subsequent exposures later in life. Ensure you are proactive in researching adequately to make informed decisions. If you only take one mindset shift from this book, let it be that YOU are responsible for making the decisions for your health and that of your loved ones. Do not allow yourself to be railroaded into acquiescing to things just because the people telling you wear white coats or carry clipboards. Having a string of letters after your name does not make you immune from mistakes or believing wrong things by virtue of biased training. Joseph Goebbels famously stated, "If you repeat a lie often enough, it becomes accepted as the truth". Do not accept things as truth without first checking for yourself to ascertain if they are correct. Iatrogenesis is real and more common than we realise.

If there is no medical reason not to, you should insist on having immediate skin-to-skin contact with your baby as soon as they are born. You want your baby to pick up YOUR skin microbiome as their first inculcation, not the *Staphylococcus* and other bacteria that can be present on the hospital equipment eagerly awaiting your infant's arrival.

Breastfeed as soon as possible to give your baby the colostrum needed to populate its gut with additional microbes to prepare it to receive your milk and to provide much-needed antibodies. Exclusively breastfeed for at least 6 months, longer if you are able, to lower the risk of Atopic development.

Source natural, non-toxic baby care products, including diapers and baby wipes. Many children can suffer terrible nappy rash, which is often just a form of dermatitis caused by a reaction to the chemicals in the products. Switching to natural organic products often resolves the problem, or when used from the outset, may prevent it from occurring in the first place.

Similarly, do your own research on vaccines so that you can make an informed decision before giving them to your child, especially if they are at a higher risk of developing eczema. '**The Truth About Vaccines**' and 'Vaxxed: From Cover-up to Catastrophe' are very informative video series backed by much research, although they have been very much maligned. There are also copious books available online to educate yourself on the alternative (usually censored) narrative. Jabbed, by Brett Wilcox, is just one example. If you decide to proceed with vaccines after examining the facts, consider spacing them out and even delaying them until after their first birthday, as per the research I quoted earlier. When I delayed my children's vaccines, the medics told me I was putting my child's health at risk, but when I asked them, "Well, if everyone else is already vaccinated, who would they catch anything from?" they did not have an answer. In all honesty, if I could turn the clock back and know then what I know now, I would not give my children any vaccines at all. But that is not medical advice. It is purely my own opinion. So, I re-iterate, do your own research from both sides of the fence. Medical censorship is becoming too similar to the 1984 Big Brother scenario, where you are not considered intelligent enough to assess facts and make an informed decision. Instead, you are treated like children and only allowed to hear one side of the story to ensure you comply with the approved narrative.

Growing Healthy Children

Do not be overly concerned with germs and bacteria. Remember I spoke about our germ-phobic lifestyles and how we are preventing our bodies from re-populating our healthy microbes by killing every perceived germ. Sodium bicarbonate, white vinegar, and essential oils are just as good at cleaning without harming the beneficial microbes.

Kids need to get dirty. Let your kids live. Let them play outside in the yard, digging soil with their hand, making mud pies, finding worms, and helping you plant organic herbs and edible plants. Getting them involved with growing food will help them to be open to trying new foods and eating a more diverse range of plant foods. Play the rainbow game with them and reward them for eating plants in all the colours of the rainbow each day.

Furthermore, increase their vitamin D intake from the sun. If you live in cooler climates, give your children vitamin D3 supplements. Regardless of where they live, every parent should consider giving their children a clean omega-3 supplement with a high dose of eicosapentaenoic acid and docosahexaenoic acid. If your child's skin is exceptionally dry despite using natural skin care products, consider giving them a weight-appropriate amount of histidine and get them tested for nutritional deficiencies, particularly those pertinent to eczema, as discussed previously. You could consult a nutritionist about histidine supplementation but bear in mind you likely know more about histidine for eczema treatment now than they do, so go armed with the reference documentation to support your arguments.

Through epigenetics, you CAN stack the odds against your children developing eczema. It begins with you changing your own epigenetic environment and continues with you managing theirs. When it comes to eczema, knowledge is power and forewarned is forearmed.

14

CONCLUSION

Congratulations on completing this book! I hope you have enjoyed reading it as much as I have enjoyed writing it. It has been a blessing to share all I have learnt with you and walk with you, albeit distantly, on your learning journey. It has taken many years of research and diagraming to reach the point where I could even consider organising everything in my head into a format I could share with others. It then took me a further year to type it all up and have it professionally edited. I am pleased with the result, and I hope you are also happy with all you have learned.

At the beginning of this book, I stated that only you could tell me whether I have succeeded in my goal to decode eczema for you and explain this complex condition in an understandable way. I hope that I have achieved it. Furthermore, I hope I have helped you gain a valuable understanding and become much better equipped to take control of your health. If this book has helped you, please let me know. You can email me directly at Carolyn@EczemaAcademy.com. You can also support me by leaving a fabulous review on Amazon.

To help other eczema sufferers find out about this book, please shout out about it on your social media platforms and in any eczema groups to which you belong. This will help me bring this helpful information to many others who need it.

Finally, for those of you who are still hungry to learn more or want to hang around with me a bit longer, here are some options for you. I will be posting FREE BONUS material on my website. I am currently writing a new chapter titled, **Is There a Spiritual Link to Eczema?** If this is a topic you are interested in finding out more about, email me to let me know and I'll add you to the wait list and let you know when it's ready. You can also subscribe to my newsletter to stay informed about the latest eczema developments and also learn more about my deep-dive eczema course if you'd like to work with me more closely.

Check out '**The Eczema Channel**' on YouTube. I regularly post new videos to share the latest eczema research and answer viewer questions about eczema. If you have questions, comment under one of the videos, and I shall endeavour to make a video with an answer for you.

I pray that God helps you and that you find healing as you take action to correct what has gone wrong. I have walked this road myself. I have felt your frustrations. I know there is a lot to action here. It takes time, effort, and money, but this is a lifestyle change, not a quick-fix solution. Some of you will implement changes quickly and, as a result, will see rapid improvements. Others will need more time to implement the changes according to your priorities. Whichever group you fall into, the important thing is to start and to keep going. If you think about the story of Noah's Ark: the cheetahs and the snails did not travel at the same pace, but they both made it into the Ark eventually.

I invested much time, effort, and money to discover all this information and then write and publish it all in this book for you. But you know what? If it helps you decode eczema and get free, it has all been worth it because you are special. You are worth it. You can do this.

APPENDIXES

References

1. Tan et al 2017. Siao Pei Tan, Simon B Brown, Christopher EM Griffiths, Richard B Weller and Neil K Gibbs "Feeding Filaggrin: Effects of L-Histidine Supplementation in Atopic Dermatitis"

2. Kezic S, O'Regan GM, Yau N et al "Levels of Filaggrin Degradation Products are Influenced by Both Filaggrin Genotype and topic Dermatitis Severity."

3. Tan SP, Abdul-Ghaffar S, Weller RB, Brown SB. "Protease-Antiprotease Imbalance May Be Linked to Potential Defects in Profilaggrin Proteolysis in Atopic Dermatitis." Br. J. Dermatol 2012:166:1137-1140 [Pubmed] [Google Scholar].

4. Kopple JD, Swendseid ME. "Evidence that Histidine is an Essential Amino Acid in Normal and Chronically Uremic Man." JClin Invest. 1875:55:881-891 (PMC free article) [PubMed] [Google Scholar]

5. Bando K, Shimotsuji T, Toyoshima H, Hayashi C, Miyai K. "Florometric Assay of Human Serum Carnosinase Activity in Normal Children, Adults and Patients with Myopathy." PMID:6517492 DOI:10.1177/004563284021006613

6. Scott IR, Harding CR, Barrett JG. "Histadine rich protein of the keratohyalin granules. Source of free amino acids, and urocanic acid and pyrrolidone carboxylic acid in the stratum corneum. Biochim Biophys Acta. 1982;719:110-117[PubMed] [Google Scholar]

7. Palmer CAN, Irvine AD, Terron-Kwiatkowski A, et al. "Common loss-of-function variants of the epidermal barrier protein filaggrin are a major predisposing factor for atopic dermatitis." 2006;38:441-446 [PubMed][Google Scholar]

8. Walling HW, Swick BL. "Update on the management of chronic eczema: new approaches and emerging treatment options." Clin Cosmet Investig Dermatol. 2010;3:99 [PMC free article] [PubMed] [Google Scholar]

9. Brown SJ et al J. Invest Dermatol 2009 Mar. "Eczema Genetics: Current state of knowledge and future goals."

10. Expression of the filaggrin gene in umbilical cord blood predicts eczema risk in infancy: A birth cohort study A.H Ziyab, S. Ewart, G.A. Lockett, H. Zhang, H. Arshad, W. Karmaus 14May 2017, https://doi.org/10.1111/cea.12956

11. Fujimura, K., Sitarik, A., Havstad, S. *et al.* "Neonatal gut microbiota associates with childhood multisensitized atopy and T cell differentiation." *Nat Med* 22, 1187–1191 (2016). https://doi.org/10.1038/nm.4176

12. Effect of probiotic *Lactobacillus* strains in children with atopic dermatitis (J Allergy Clin Immunol 2003;111:389-95.)

13. Probiotics Supplementation During Pregnancy or Infancy for the Prevention of Atopic Dermatitis: A Meta-analysis Pelucchi, Claudio, et al. "Review Article: Probiotics Supplementation During Pregnancy or Infancy for the Prevention of Atopic Dermatitis: A Meta-Analysis." *Epidemiology*, vol. 23, no. 3, 2012, pp. 402–414., www.jstor.org/stable/23214270. Accessed 24 Apr. 2020.

14. Hornerin is a component of the epidermal cornified cell envelopes. The FASEB Journal fj.10-168658 Published January 31 2011 Julie Henry, Chiung-Yueh Hsu, Marek Haftek, Rachida Nachat, Heleen D. de Koning, Isabelle Gardinal-Galera, Kiyotaka Hitomi, Stefana Balica, Catherine Jean-Decoster, Anne-Marie Schmitt, Carle Paul, Guy Serre, and Michel Simon

15. Loss-of-Function Mutations in the *Filaggrin* Gene and Allergic Contact Sensitization to Nickel-Science Direct Natalija Novak Hansjörg Baurecht Torsten Schäfer Elke Rodriguez Stefan Wagenpfeil Norman Klopp Joachim Heinrich Heidrun Behrendt Johannes Ring Erich Wichmann ThomasIllig Stephan Weidinger

16. Eczema: Pathophysiology updated May 2013 Worldallergy.org Prof. Dr. Ulf Darsow, Prof. Dr. Kilian Eyerich, Prof. Dr. Johannes Ring https://www.worldallergy.org/education-and-programs/education/allergic-disease-resource-center/professionals/eczema-pathophysiology

17. Science Direct T-cell subsets (Th1 versus Th2) Author Sergio Romagnani

18. Aluminum based vaccines can cause aluminum allergy in DTP vaccines ncbi-nlm.nih.gov – Neilson AO et al Ugeskr Laegar 1992

19. MDedge.com New worldwide atopic dermatitis survey

20. Biotin production by Bifidobacterium 1993 Hiroko Noda, Noriko Akasaka, and Masahiro Ohsugi

21. Early-Life Antibiotic-Driven Dysbiosis Leads to Dysregulated Vaccine Immune Responses in Mice Miriam Anne Lynn, Damon John Tumes, Jocelyn Mei Choo, Anastasia Sribnaia, Stephen James Blake, Lex Ee Xiang Leong, Graeme Paul Young, Helen Siobhan Marshall, Steve Lodewijk Wesselingh, Geraint Berian Rogers, David John Lynn PMID: 29746836 DOI: 10.1016/j.chom.2018.04.009

22. Nevilde Maria Riselo sales, Patricia Barbosa Pelegrini and Maria Clara da Silva Goersch, "Nutrigenomics: Definitionsand Advances of This New Science." Journal of Nutrition and Metabolism (2014) 202759 https://doi.org/10.1155/2014/202759

23. Clinical immunology The effect of *Zingiber officinale* R. rhizomes (ginger) on plasma pro-inflammatory cytokine levels in well-trained male endurance runners. Farzad Zehsaz, Negin Farhangi, Lamia Mirheidari. *(Centr Eur J Immunol 2014; 39 (2): 174–180),* DOI: https://doi.org/10.5114/ceji.2014.43719, Online publish date: 2014/06/27

24. *Nutrients* 2018, *10*(11), 1567; https://doi.org/10.3390/nu10111567 Ginger Extract Ameliorates Obesity and Inflammation via Regulating MicroRNA-21/132 Expression and AMPK Activation in White Adipose Tissue, S. Kim, M-S. Lee, S. Jung, H-Y Son, S Park, B. Kang, S-Y Kim, IH Kim, C-T Kim, Y Kim.

25. https://bio.libretexts.org/Bookshelves/Introductory_and_General_Biology/Book%3A_Introductory_Biology_(CK-12)/13%3A_Human_Biology/13.74%3A_Skin

26. Journal of Family Medicine and Primary Care. Iatrogenesis: A review on nature, extent, and distribution of healthcare hazards. Rafia Farooq Peer and Nadeem Sahbir PMCID:PMC6060929 PMID:30090769

27. Informed Health.org [internet]. Cologne, Germany: Institute for Quality and Efficiency in Health Care (IQWiG); 2006- How Does Skin Work? 2009 Sep 28 [Updated 2019 Apr 11]

28. Exp Diabetes Res doi:10.1155/2012/128694 PMCID:PMC3415238 PMID:22899900 Xing Liu, Chang-Bin Sun, Ting-Tong Yang, Da Li, Chun-Yan Li, Yan-Jie Tian, Ming Guo, Yu Cao, and Shi-Sheng Zhou

29. Immunol Rev.2011 Jul;242(1):233-246. Doi:10.1111/j.1600-065X.2011.01027.x PMCID:PMC3122139 NIHM-SID:NIHMS291015 PMID:21682749

30. Structure of normal skin; Author Dr.Anthony Yung, Dermatologist, Waikato District Health Board, Hamilton, New Zealand 2007 DermNet NZ.org

31. Association between atopic dermatitis and auto-immune disorders in US adults and children: A cross-sectional study Narla S, Silverberg JI. J Am Academy Dermatology. 2019;80:382-389. Doi;10.2016/j.jaad.2018.09.025

32. *(JAMA,* July 26, 2000—Vol 284, No. 4) https://jamanetwork.com/journals/jama/article-abstract/192908?redirect=true)

33. https://www.hopkinsmedicine.org/news/media/releases/study_suggests_medical_errors_now_third_leading_cause_of_death_in_the_us

34. Ha-Jung Kim, Young-Joon Kim, Seung-Hwa Lee, Jinho Yu, Se Kyoo Jeong, Soo-Jong Hong, Effects of Lactobacillus Rhamnosous on allergic march model by suppressing Th2, Th17, and TSLP responses via CD4+CD25+Foxp3+ Tregs, Clinical Immunology, Volume 153, Issue 1, 2014, Pages 178-186, ISSN 1521-6616, https://doi.org/10.1016/j.clim.2014.04.008. (http://www.sciencedirect.com/science/article/pii/S1521661614001156)

35. Clinicaltrials.gov The Effects of Aspirin and Acetaminophen on the Stomach in Health Volunteers University of Illinois, January 16, 2018

36. Megan Clapp et al., "Gut Microbiota's Effect on Mental Health: The Gut-Brain Axis," Clinics and Practice 7, no.4 (2017):987, https://doi.org/10.4081/cp.2017.987

37. M. Nazmul Huda et al., "Stool Microbiota and Vaccine Response of Infants," Pediatrics 134, no. 2 (2014): e362-72, https://doi.org/10.1542/peds.2013-3937

38. Vitamin A deficiency exacerbates extrinsic atopic dermatitis development by potentiating type 2 helper T cell-type inflammation and mast cell activation June 2020 Clinical & Experimental Allergy 50(8) DOI: 10.1111/cea.13687

39. Zaniboni MC, Samorano LP, Orfali RL, Aoki V. Skin barrier in atopic dermatitis: beyond filaggrin. *An Bras Dermatol.* 2016;91(4):472-478. doi:10.1590/abd1806-4841.20164412

40. The Involvement of the JAK-STAT signalling pathway in chronic inflammatory skin disease atopic dermatitis. JAKSTAT. 2013 Jul1;2(3):e24137 doi:10.4161/jkst.24137 PMCID:PMC3772104 PMID:24069552

41. Mechanisms of Regulatory t-cell suppression – a diverse arsenal for a moving target- doi:10.1111/j.1365-2567.2008.02813.x PMCID: PMC2434375 PMID: 18346152 Immunology. 2008 May: 124(1): 13-22.

42. Rahnama P, Montazeri A, Huseini HF, Kianbakht S, Naseri M. Effect of Zingiber officinale R. rhizomes (ginger) on pain relief in primary dysmenorrhea: a placebo randomized trial. *BMC Complement Altern Med.* 2012;12:92. Published 2012 Jul 10. doi:10.1186/1472-6882-12-92

43. https://www.ncbi.nlm.nih.gov/pmc/articles/PMC4828648/ Probiotics and Atopic Dermatitis: An Overview

44. [Frontiers in Bioscience 16, 1768-1786, January 1, 2011] 1768 Amino acid metabolism in intestinal bacteria: links between gut ecology and host health Zhao-Lai Dai1 , Guoyao Wu2, 3, Wei-Yun Zhu1

45. Oliphant, K., Allen-Vercoe, E. Macronutrient metabolism by the human gut microbiome: major fermentation by-products and their impact on host health. *Microbiome* 7, 91 (2019). https://doi.org/10.1186/s40168-019-0704-8

46. Neis EPJG, Dejong CHC, Rensen SS. The Role of Microbial Amino Acid Metabolism in Host Metabolism. *Nutrients*. 2015; 7(4):2930-2946. https://doi.org/10.3390/nu7042930

47. Bentham Science Publishers DOI: https://doi.org/10.2174/187152810792231896 Lactobacillus rhamnosus cell lysate in the management of resistant childhood atopic eczema

48. *Mangifera indica* L. extract (Vimang) and mangiferin reduce the airway inflammation and Th2 cytokines in murine model of allergic asthma Dagmar García Rivera, Ivones Hernández, Nelson Merino, Yilian Luque, Alina Álvarez, Yanet Martín, Aylin Amador, Lauro Nuevas, René Delgado, https://onlinelibrary.wiley.com/doi/abs/10.1111/j.2042-7158.2011.01328.x

49. Anti-allergic properties of Mangifera indica L. extract (Vimang) and contribution of its glucosylxanthone mangiferin, Dagmar García Rivera Ivones Hernández Balmaseda Alina Álvarez León Belkis Cancio Hernández Lucía Márquez Montiel Gabino Garrido René Delgado Hernández Salvatore Cuzzocrea https://onlinelibrary.wiley.com/doi/abs/10.1211/jpp.58.3.0014

50. Chirayath RB, A AV, Jayakumar R, Biswas R, Vijayachandran LS. Development of Mangifera indica leaf extract incorporated carbopol hydrogel and its antibacterial efficacy against Staphylococcus aureus. Colloids Surf B Biointerfaces. 2019 Jun 1;178:377-384. doi: 10.1016/j.colsurfb.2019.03.034. Epub 2019 Mar 15. PMID: 30903976.

51. Mangiferin glycethosomes as a new potential adjuvant for the treatment of psoriasis, M Pleguezuelos-Villa, Octavio Diez-Sales, Maria Letizia Manca, Maria Manconi, Amparo Ruiz Sauri, Elvira Escribano-Ferrer, Amparo Nácher, Affiliations expand, PMID: 31751638 DOI: 10.1016/j.ijpharm.2019.118844

52. Holeček M. Histidine in Health and Disease: Metabolism, Physiological Importance, and Use as a Supplement. Nutrients. 2020;12(3):848. Published 2020 Mar 22. doi:10.3390/nu12030848

53. Laura Maintz, Natalija Novak, Histamine and histamine intolerance, The American Journal of Clinical Nutrition, Volume 85, Issue 5, May 2007, Pages 1185–1196, https://doi.org/10.1093/ajcn/85.5.1185

54. Yee, S.W., Lin, L., Merski, M. et al. Prediction and validation of enzyme and transporter off-targets for metformin. J Pharmacokinet Pharmacodyn 42, 463–475 (2015). https://doi.org/10.1007/s10928-015-9436-y

55. https://www.greenmedinfo.com/blog/200-clinically-confirmed-reasons-not-eat-wheat

56. Militaryhistorynow.com Fatal Errors – The Worst Friendly Fire Incidents of World War Two.

57. Pizzino G, Irrera N, Cucinotta M, et al. Oxidative Stress: Harms and Benefits for Human Health. Oxid Med Cell Longev. 2017;2017:8416763. doi:10.1155/2017/8416763

58. MDPI and ACS Style Zhang, F.; Wang, D. The Pattern of microRNA Binding Site Distribution. Genes 2017, 8, 296. https://doi.org/10.3390/genes8110296

59. Yang SN, Hsieh CC, Kuo HF, et al. The effects of environmental toxins on allergic inflammation. Allergy Asthma Immunol Res. 2014;6(6):478-484. doi:10.4168/aair.2014.6.6.47

60. Levander OA. Lead toxicity and nutritional deficiencies. Environ Health Perspect. 1979 Apr;29:115-25. doi: 10.1289/ehp.7929115. PMID: 510231; PMCID: PMC1637366.

61. Stone KD, Prussin C, Metcalfe DD. IgE, mast cells, basophils, and eosinophils. J Allergy Clin Immunol. 2010;125(2 Suppl 2):S73-S80. doi:10.1016/j.jaci.2009.11.017

62. https://www.merckmanuals.com/home/immune-disorders/allergic-reactions-and-other-hypersensitivity-disorders/exercise-induced-allergic-reactions

63. Minty B. Food-dependent exercise-induced anaphylaxis. *Can Fam Physician*. 2017;63(1):42-43.

64. Kim K. Influences of Environmental Chemicals on Atopic Dermatitis. *Toxicol Res*. 2015;31(2):89-96. doi:10.5487/TR.2015.31.2.089

65. Nicolson GL. Mitochondrial Dysfunction and Chronic Disease: Treatment With Natural Supplements. Integr Med (Encinitas). 2014;13(4):35-43.

66. https://lpi.oregonstate.edu/mic/dietary-factors/coenzyme-Q10

67. https://ods.od.nih.gov/factsheets/Niacin-HealthProfessional/

68. Küllenberg D, Taylor LA, Schneider M, Massing U. Health effects of dietary phospholipids. Lipids Health Dis. 2012;11:3. Published 2012 Jan 5. doi:10.1186/1476-511X-11-3

69. https://www.atopona.sk/wp-content/uploads/2020/06/ATO-097-Serum-heavymetal-levels-are-associated-with-asthma-allergic-rhinitis-atopic-dermatitis-allergic-multimorbidity-and-airflow-obstruction.pdf

70. Seulbi Lee, Sung Kyun Park, Hyesook Park, Woojoo Lee, Jung Hyun Kwon, Yun-Chul Hong, Mina Ha, Yangho Kim, Boeun Lee, Eunhee Ha, Prenatal heavy metal exposures and atopic dermatitis with gender difference in 6-month-old infants using multipollutant analysis, Environmental Research, Volume 195, 2021, 110865, ISSN 0013-9351, https://doi.org/10.1016/j.envres.2021.110865. (https://www.sciencedirect.com/science/article/pii/S0013935121001596)

71. The influence of breast and artificial feeding on infantile eczema. 10.1016/S0022-3476(36)80058-4 Journal of Pediatrics 1936 Vol.9 pp.223-225 Grulee, C. G. ; Sanford, H. N.

72. Combined effects of prenatal medication use and delivery type are associated with eczema at age 2 years https://doi.org/10.1111/cea.12467

73. Robin Mesnage, Nicolas Defarge, Joël Spiroux de Vendômois, Gilles-Eric Séralini, "Major Pesticides Are More Toxic to Human Cells Than Their Declared Active Principles", *BioMed*

Research International, vol. 2014, Article ID 179691, 8 pages, 2014. https://doi.org/10.1155/2014/179691

74. The impact of food additives, artifcial sweeteners and domestic hygiene products on the human gut microbiome and its fibre fermentation capacity European Journal of Nutrition (2020) 59:3213–3230 https://doi.org/10.1007/s00394-019-02161-8

75. Sato S. Iron deficiency: structural and microchemical changes in hair, nails, and skin. Seminars in Dermatology. 1991 Dec;10(4):313-319.

76. Effect of lipid peroxidation, antioxidants, macro minerals and trace elements on eczema Arch Dermatol Res (2015) 307:617–623 DOI 10.1007/s00403-015-1570-2

77. Fish oil supplementation alters levels of lipid mediators of inflammation in microenvironment of acute human wounds Jodi C. McDaniel PhD Karen Massey PhD Anna Nicolaou PhD First published: 01 March 2011 https://doi.org/10.1111/j.1524-475X.2010.00659.x

78. Anti-inflammatory Properties of Curcumin, a Major Constituent of Curcuma longa: A Review of Preclinical and Clinical Research Julie S* Jurenka, MT(ASCP) Alternative Medicine Review Volume 14, Number 2 2009

79. Rachel Leproult, Georges Copinschi, Orfeu Buxton, Eve Van Cauter, Sleep Loss Results in an Elevation of Cortisol Levels the Next Evening, *Sleep*, Volume 20, Issue 10, October 1997, Pages 865–870, https://doi.org/10.1093/sleep/20.10.865

80. Ekstedt, Mirjam BNSci; Åkerstedt, Torbjörn PhD; Söderström, Marie MSci Microarousals During Sleep Are Associated With Increased Levels of Lipids, Cortisol, and Blood Pressure, Psychosomatic Medicine: November 2004 - Volume 66 - Issue 6 - p 925-931 doi: 10.1097/01.psy.0000145821.25453.f7

81. Kenneth P. Wright, Amanda L. Drake, Danielle J. Frey, Monika Fleshner, Christopher A. Desouza, Claude Gronfier, Charles A. Czeisler, Influence of sleep deprivation and circadian misalignment on cortisol, inflammatory markers, and

cytokine balance, Brain, Behavior, and Immunity, Volume 47, 2015, Pages 24-34, ISSN 0889-1591, https://doi.org/10.1016/j.bbi.2015.01.004,(https://www.sciencedirect.com/science/article/pii/S0889159115000069)

82. Postepy Hig Med Dosw (online), 2016; 70: 380-391 e-ISSN 1732-2693 https://naturalsolutions.nz/articles/Frankincense-therapeutic-properties-2016.pdf

83. Genkinger JM, Koushik A (2007) Meat Consumption and Cancer Risk. PLoS Med 4(12): e345. https://doi.org/10.1371/journal.pmed.0040345

84. Campos FA, FloresH, Underwood BA. Effect of an infection on vitamin A status of children as measured by the relative dose response) RDR.Am J Clin Nutr. 1987 Jul:46(1):91-4. Doi: 10.1093/ajcn/46.1.91. PMID:3604975

85. Vitamin A deficiency and its consequences. A field guide to detection and control 3rd edition. Alfred Sommer. World Health Organization

86. Oschman JL, Chevalier G, Brown R. The effects of grounding (earthing) on inflammation, the immune response, wound healing, and prevention and treatment of chronic inflammatory and autoimmune diseases. *J Inflamm Res.* 2015;8:83-96. Published 2015 Mar 24. doi:10.2147/JIR.S69656

87. Tarasov EA, Blinov DV, Zimovina UV, Sandakova EA. [Magnesium deficiency and Stress: Issues of their relationship, diagnostic tests, and approaches to therapy]. Ter Arkh. 2015;87(9):10.17116/terarkh2015879114-122.PMID:26591563

88. Ehrhardt Proksch MD, PhD, Hans-Peter Nissen PhD, Markus Bremgartner MD, Colin Urquhart PhD Bathing in a Magnesium-rich Dead Sea salt solution improves skin barrier function, enhances skin hydration, and reduces inflammation in atopic dry skin https://doi.org/10.1111/j.1365-4632.2005.02079.x

89. Ivana Buric, Miguel Farias, Jonathan Jong, Christopher Mee, Inti A Brazil. What Is the Molecular Signature of Mind–Body Interventions? A Systematic Review of Gene Expression

Changes Induced by Meditation and Related Practices Front. Immunol., 16 June 2017 | https://doi.org/10.3389/fimmu.2017.00670

90. Lee YL, Su HJ, Sheu HM, Yu HS, Guo YL. Traffic-related air pollution, climate, and prevalence of eczema in Taiwanese school children. J Invest Dermatol. 2008 Oct;128(10):2412-20. doi: 10.1038/jid.2008.110. Epub 2008 May 1. PMID: 18449213.

91. Kantor R, Silverberg JI. Environmental risk factors and their role in the management of atopic dermatitis. *Expert Rev Clin Immunol*. 2017;13(1):15-26. doi:10.1080/174466 6X.2016.1212660

92. Morgenstern V, Zutavern A, Cyrys J, Brockow I, Koletzko S, Krämer U, Behrendt H, Herbarth O, von Berg A, Bauer CP, Wichmann HE, Heinrich J; GINI Study Group; LISA Study Group. Atopic diseases, allergic sensitization, and exposure to traffic-related air pollution in children. Am J Respir Crit Care Med. 2008 Jun 15;177(12):1331-7. doi: 10.1164/rccm.200701-036OC. Epub 2008 Mar 12. PMID: 18337595.

93. Jedrychowski W, Perera F, Maugeri U, Mrozek-Budzyn D, Miller RL, Flak E, Mroz E, Jacek R, Spengler JD. Effects of prenatal and perinatal exposure to fine air pollutants and maternal fish consumption on the occurrence of infantile eczema. Int Arch Allergy Immunol. 2011;155(3):275-81. doi: 10.1159/000320376. Epub 2011 Feb 3. PMID: 21293147; PMCID: PMC3047761.

94. Just AC, Whyatt RM, Perzanowski MS, Calafat AM, Perera FP, Goldstein IF, Chen Q, Rundle AG, Miller RL. Prenatal exposure to butylbenzyl phthalate and early eczema in an urban cohort. Environ Health Perspect. 2012 Oct;120(10):1475-80. doi: 10.1289/ehp.1104544. Epub 2012 Jun 26. PMID: 22732598; PMCID: PMC3491925.

95. Kim J, Kim EH, Oh I, Jung K, Han Y, Cheong HK, Ahn K. Symptoms of atopic dermatitis are influenced by outdoor air pollution. J Allergy Clin Immunol. 2013 Aug;132(2):495-8. e1. doi: 10.1016/j.jaci.2013.04.019. Epub 2013 Jun 12. PMID: 23763977.

96. Lee JH, Suh J, Kim EH, et al. Surveillance of home environment in children with atopic dermatitis: a questionnaire survey. *Asia Pac Allergy*. 2012;2(1):59-66. doi:10.5415/apallergy.2012.2.1.59

97. Yi O, Kwon HJ, Kim H, Ha M, Hong SJ, Hong YC, Leem JH, Sakong J, Lee CG, Kim SY, Kang D. Effect of environmental tobacco smoke on atopic dermatitis among children in Korea. Environ Res. 2012 Feb;113:40-5. doi: 10.1016/j.envres.2011.12.012. Epub 2012 Jan 21. PMID: 22264877.

98. Effects of Components Derived from Diesel Exhaust Particles on Lung Physiology Related to Antigen Ken-Ichiro Inoue,Hirohisa Takano,Rie Yanagisawa,Miho Sakurai,Satomi Abe,Shin Yoshino,Kouya Yamaki &Toshikazu Yoshikawa Pages 403-412 | Published online: 08 Oct 2008 Download citation https://doi.org/10.1080/08923970701675002

99. Wang I.J., Guo Y.L., Lin T.J., Chen P.C., Wu Y.N. GSTM1, GSTP1, prenatal smoke exposure, and atopic dermatitis. *Ann. Allergy Asthma Immunol.* (2010);105:124–129. doi: 10.1016/j. anai.2010.04.017. [PubMed] [CrossRef] [Google Scholar]

100.Eberlein-König B, Przybilla B, Kühnl P, Pechak J, Gebefügi I, Kleinschmidt J, Ring J. Influence of airborne nitrogen dioxide or formaldehyde on parameters of skin function and cellular activation in patients with atopic eczema and control subjects. J Allergy Clin Immunol. 1998 Jan;101(1 Pt 1):141-3. doi: 10.1016/S0091-6749(98)70212-X. PMID: 9449520.

101.Huss-Marp J, Eberlein-König B, Breuer K, Mair S, Ansel A, Darsow U, Krämer U, Mayer E, Ring J, Behrendt H. Influence of short-term exposure to airborne Der p 1 and volatile organic compounds on skin barrier function and dermal blood flow in patients with atopic eczema and healthy individuals. Clin Exp Allergy. 2006 Mar;36(3):338-45. doi: 10.1111/j.1365-2222.2006.02448.x. PMID: 16499645.

102.Effectiveness of Commercial and Homemade Washing Agents in Removing Pesticide Residues on and in Apples. Tianxi Yang, Jeffery Doherty, Bin Zhao, Amanda J. Kinchla, John M. Clark, and Lili He, J. Agric. Food Chem, 2017, 65, 97/acs.jafc.7b03118

103. Correlation of Tissue Antibodies and Food Immune Reactivity in Randomly Selected Patient Specimens Jama Lambert1 * and Aristo Vojdani J Clin Cell Immunol 2017, 8:5 DOI: 10.4172/2155-9899.1000521

104. Society for General Microbiology. "Essential oils to fight superbugs." ScienceDaily. ScienceDaily, 4 April 2010. <www.sciencedaily.com/releases/2010/03/100330210942.htm>.

105. The Use of Shea Butter as an Emollient for Eczema Essengue Belibi, S; Stechschulte, D; Olson, N.Journal of Allergy and Clinical Immunology, suppl. Supplement; St. Louis Vol. 123, Iss. 2, (Feb 2009): S41. DOI:10.1016/j.jaci.2008.12.1100

106. Atopic eczema and domestic water hardness https://doi.org/10.1016/S0140-6736(98)01402-0 The Lancet volume 352, issue 9127

107. Interactions between domestic water hardness, infant swimming and atopy in the development of childhood eczema https://doi.org/10.1016/j.envres.2012.04.013

108. Bamji E, Bamji N. Severe dermatitis and "biological" detergents. Br Med J. 1970;1(5696):629. doi:10.1136/bmj.1.5696.629

109. Addressing the Challenge of Topical Steroid Withdrawal BY PETER A. LIO, MD http://v2.practicaldermatology.com/pdfs/PD0915_clinfocus.pdf

110. Scherrer MA, Rocha VB, Andrade AR. Contact dermatitis to methylisothiazolinone. *An Bras Dermatol.* 2015;90(6):912-914. doi:10.1590/abd1806-4841.20153992

111. https://www.fiercepharma.com/drug-delivery/what-heart-safety-concern-doctors-like-incyte-s-ruxolitinib-atopic-dermatitis-cream

112. Effect Of Essential Oils On Some Pathogens That Cause Eczema Meryem Karaçam, Durmuş Alpaslan Kaya* Mustafa Kemal University, Faculty of Agriculture, Department of Field Crops http://icams.ro/icamsresurse/2020/files/lucrari/II_biomaterials_biotechnologies_13.pdf

113. ASEA https://doi.org/10.1067/mic.2000.105287 American Journal of Infection Control Microbicidal activity of MDI-P against *Candida albicans, Staphylococcus aureus, Pseudomonas aeruginosa,* and *Legionella pneumophila*

114. https://pubmed.ncbi.nlm.nih.gov/16930802/ L-Theanine reduces psychological and physiological stress responses

115. https://www.sciencedirect.com/science/article/abs/pii/S00916674904033743 Dermatitis caused by indoor mold exposure W.J. Rockwell J. Santilli DOI: https://doi.org/10.1016/j.jaci.2004.12.118

116. "Imagine You Are an Aluminum Atom" by Christopher Exley Ph.D.., FRSB

117. Which aeroallergens are associated with eczema severity? K. L. E. Hon,T. F. Leung,M. C. A. Lam,K. Y. Wong,C. M. Chow,T. F. Fok,P. C. Ng First published: 08 April 2007 https://doi.org/10.1111/j.1365-2230.2007.02420.x

118. Mite elimination – clinical effect on eczema P. S. Friedmann,B. B. Tan First published: 30 December 2008 https://doi.org/10.1111/j.1398-9995.1998.tb05007.x

119. Home environment and suspected atopic eczema in Japanese infants: The Osaka Maternal and Child Health Study, Yoshihiro Miyake, Department of Public Health, Faculty of Medicine, Fukuoka University, Fukuoka 814-0180, Japan https://onlinelibrary.wiley.com/doi/abs/10.1111/j.1399-3038.2007.00545.x

120. Associations between home dampness-related exposures and childhood eczema among 13,335 preschool children in Shanghai, China: A cross-sectional study, https://www.sciencedirect.com/science/article/abs/pii/S0013935115301699

121. https://www.researchgate.net/profile/Francisco-Guillen-Grima/publication/6254402_Role_of_the_home_environment_in_rhinoconjunctivitis_and_eczema_in_schoolchildren_in_Pamplona_Spain/links/0c960517f6b274068c000000/Role-of-the-home-environment-in-rhinoconjunctivitis-and-eczema-in-schoolchildren-in-Pamplona-Spain.pdf

122. Adverse health effects in children associated with moisture and mold observations in houses. Outi M. Koskinen,Tuula M. Husman,Teija M. Meklin &Aino I. Nevalainen Pages 143-156 | Published online: 21 Jul 2010 https://www.tandfonline.com/doi/abs/10.1080/09603129973281

123. Mold-sensitivity in children with moderate-severe asthma is associated with HLA-DR and HLA-DQA. P. Knutsen,H. M. Vijay,V. Kumar,B. Kariuki,L. A. Santiago,R. Graff,J. D. Wofford,M. R. Shah, https://onlinelibrary.wiley.com/doi/abs/10.1111/j.1398-9995.2010.02382.x

124. Mold elicits atopic dermatitis by reactive oxygen species: Epidemiology and mechanism studies, Ha-JungKimaE-unLeebcSeung-HwaLeeaMi-JinKangaSoo-JongHong-bc, https://www.sciencedirect.com/science/article/abs/pii/S1521661615300103

125. Vitamin D3 attenuates Th2 responses to Aspergillus fumigatus mounted by CD4+ T cells from cystic fibrosis patients with allergic bronchopulmonary aspergillosis, James L. Kreindler,1 Chad Steele,2 Nikki Nguyen,3 Yvonne R. Chan,4 Joseph M. Pilewski,4 John F. Alcorn,1 Yatin M. Vyas,1 Shean J. Aujla,1 Peter Finelli,3 Megan Blanchard,1 Steven F. Zeigler,5 Alison Logar,1 Elizabeth Hartigan,1 Marcia Kurs-Lasky,6 Howard Rockette,6 Anuradha Ray,4 and Jay K. Kolls1,3, https://www.jci.org/articles/view/42388

126. T-Cell Subsets (TH1 vs TH2) Sergio Romagnani, https://doi.org/10.1016/S1081-1206(10)62426-X Annals of Allergy, Asthma & Immunology, Volume 85, Issue 1, July 2000, Pages 9-18, 21